MY YEARS AS AN ALZHEIMER'S CAREGIVER:

transcending loss by nurturing spirit

Lyla Yastion

First published in 2025 by Blossom Spring Publishing
MY YEARS AS AN ALZHEIMER'S CAREGIVER:
transcending loss by nurturing spirit
Copyright © 2025 Lyla Yastion
ISBN 978-1-0683266-8-4
E: admin@blossomspringpublishing.com
W: www.blossomspringpublishing.com

For All Those Living with
Alzheimer's Disease and Their Caregivers

There are two aspects in Nature: the perishable and the imperishable. All life in this world belongs to the former; the unchanging element belongs to the latter.

The Bhagavad Gita

Table of Contents

Acknowledgements

This book is based in part on journal entries I kept for the six years in which I cared for my husband, Edward, who had Alzheimer's disease. Journaling provided the opportunity to record what I was learning about the disease from the study of brain science and the observation of my husband's increasing cognitive decline. It was also a means of unloading and digesting the emotional undercurrent that accompanied the unfolding of this new development in our relationship. I was Edward's sole caregiver. There were times, especially in the final year of Edward's life, when I had to count on our family for help. I want to express my gratitude for the indispensable support of our two sons, John and James, as well as their wives, Magda and Ronnie respectively. Even as they felt the emotional burden of watching Edward's mental deterioration, they offered me both steadiness and empathy.

I decided, after Edward's death, to write this book in his honor. I wanted to help fellow caregivers in their journeys by recounting my own experiences and the lessons I learned, often from the mistakes I made. Although the main case study is of my husband, Edward, I have included the stories of two friends: Michael and David. Their wives had Alzheimer's disease. Michael's wife, Eileen, lived with Alzheimer's for ten years. David's wife, Karen, had Alzheimer's for four years. I thank both men for their willingness to be interviewed and share their experiences. I appreciate the honest, in-depth recounting of their journeys as they navigated the labyrinth of Alzheimer's disease with their wives. I would also like to acknowledge the input of two other people who helped me better

1

understand the disease, how it presents, and how it progresses: Rev. Diane Epstein, an interfaith minister and chaplain at Hudson Valley Hospice, and Dr. Jodi Friedman, geriatrician at The Center for Healthy Aging at Northern Dutchess Hospital, Rhinebeck, N.Y. Two important resources in both research and practical assistance were the Alzheimer's Association and the Hospice Foundation.

I want to thank my friend, Susan Slotnik, for her indispensable collaboration in bringing the book to its final shape. Susan is a writer as well as a dancer, teacher, and painter. She has a keen eye and was willing to read the manuscript, as it went through several drafts, and offer editorial advice. Her dogged reminder to keep the journal entries real and true, not leaving out unpleasant or difficult moments, was invaluable.

The two Japanese brush paintings displayed in the book were painted by my husband, Edward. I want to thank David for allowing me to also include one of the many pieces of art which he and his wife, Karen, collaborated on during her illness.

The following publishers and copyright holders have generously given permission to use excerpts from the following sources:

From *You Are Here: Discovering the Magic of the Present Moment* by Thich Nhat Hanh. Copyright © 2001 Éditions Dangles – Saint-Jean-de-Braye (France) and © 2001 by Unified Buddhist Church, Inc. Reprinted by arrangement with The Permissions Company, LLC on behalf of Shambhala Publications Inc., Boulder, Colorado, www.shambhala.com.

From *Fear and Trembling* by Soren Kierkegaard published by Penguin Classics. Translation Copyright © Alastair Hannay, 1985. Reprinted by permission of Penguin Books Limited.

All other permissions are acknowledged in the endnotes.

Biographical Note

As our story unfolds, I would like you, as reader, to have at least a mental picture of the main character of this book: my husband, Edward. He is 6 feet 1 inches, lean and handsome in a rugged kind of way, with Slavic features such as high cheekbones and deep-set, hazel eyes which reflect his Polish/Ukrainian descent. His smile is disarming and one of the first things that swept me off my feet fifty-five years ago. Edward has an even temperament. He is a gentle-man, modest about his accomplishments.

Edward was born on February 1st, 1934, the second son of an immigrant family who came to the United States from Poland in the 1920s and settled in the southside of Pittsburgh. His father worked in the coal mines for a dollar a day, his mother in the soap factory. As a young man, Edward was not passionate about academics. He finished high school at a vocational school where he learned carpentry, a skill which he would master later in life.

Edward entered the Army as a nineteen-year-old; his two-year stint in the Armed Forces was during the Korean War. He had the good fortune to be chosen for the presidential honor guard in Washington D.C., instead of being sent to Korea like some of his buddies. He was persuaded by a fellow soldier, who had experience as an actor, to attend college when he left the Army and major in drama. Edward took his friend's advice, earned an exemplary recommendation from his commanding officer, and was accepted at Carnegie Mellon University. He graduated with a BFA in Theatre Arts. Edward was the first in his family to get a college education.

Edward's early career was in the theatre. We met at Herbert Berghof Studio in New York City where we were both studying acting. A romantic relationship quickly developed. We were married ten months later. We rented a tiny apartment in the East Village which was the hub of the hippie culture in the 1960s. Edward totally renovated the apartment. A theatre friend of his called the diminutive space Queen Victoria's closet. With mutual friends we established a summer stock company in Rhode Island. For two years we put on plays, which were well received. However, as anyone in theatre knows, it's hard to make a living at it. So, theatre was replaced by Edward's establishment of a cabinet making business on 20th St. in New York City. He became a sought-after master carpenter. Perhaps it was his agile movements – those of a dancer (he taught ballroom dancing at Arthur Murray Studio before I knew him) – that made watching him work such a pleasure. When I became pregnant with our first son, John, we moved from E. 9th St. and joined three other families in purchasing a brownstone on the upper west side. Edward was in heaven refurbishing the parquet floors and cherry wood fireplaces. His business, plus a few good real estate purchases, provided a steady income as our family grew once more with the birth of our second son, James.

Besides his family, Edward's great love was his connection to what spiritual seekers call the Teaching or the Work. He and I found the Teaching at The School of Practical Philosophy in New York City where we attended classes and offered service for many years. The School was founded in London, England by Leon McLaren. Branches of the School exist all over the world. It is set up as a traditional educational institution with lower, middle, and upper school levels. Everyone who comes to the

School is a student of philosophy first. After several terms, a second line of work is offered – service in some capacity. Students who serve in the capacity of teachers are called tutors. All service is voluntary.

The School teaches the art of presence, of staying awake and attentive to the moment, so that one can respond to whatever the moment brings in an effective, selfless manner. The intention is to dedicate one's actions to God, to the Absolute. The material used in classes is eclectic, gleaned from the spiritual teachings of East and West, with a leaning towards the East and Advaita Vedanta. Initiation into mantra meditation is offered to students. Meditation is considered the backbone of spiritual practice.

Over the forty-three years of Edward's participation as a student and tutor he was given several leadership roles. One role was team leader, in charge of training and execution of physical work. The latter is an important vehicle for students to learn the art of attention, how to connect mind to body in executing a physical task with dexterity and precision. Edward's kindness, humility, and commitment to teaching this art of attention in physical work was and is recounted with appreciation by students who were in his care. On the next page is a sign of instructions for work that is still hanging in the shop area of the School's retreat house in Wallkill, NY.

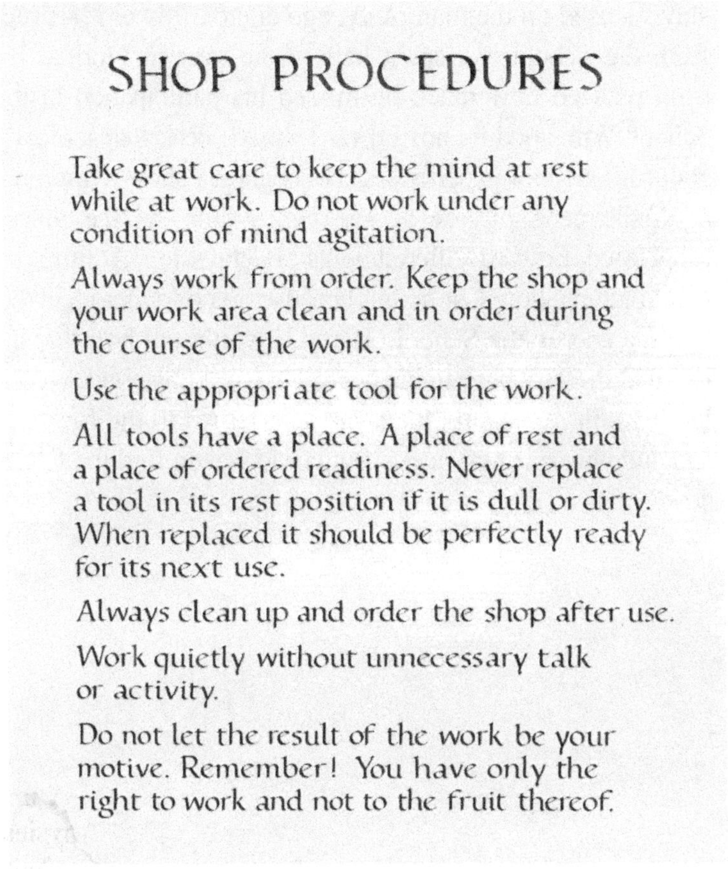

SHOP PROCEDURES

Take great care to keep the mind at rest while at work. Do not work under any condition of mind agitation.

Always work from order. Keep the shop and your work area clean and in order during the course of the work.

Use the appropriate tool for the work.

All tools have a place. A place of rest and a place of ordered readiness. Never replace a tool in its rest position if it is dull or dirty. When replaced it should be perfectly ready for its next use.

Always clean up and order the shop after use.

Work quietly without unnecessary talk or activity.

Do not let the result of the work be your motive. Remember! You have only the right to work and not to the fruit thereof.

Image 1: Shop Procedures, The School of Practical Philosophy, Wallkill, NY, used with permission

Another leadership role Edward assumed was head of meditation. It will be evident in the chronicling of his experience with Alzheimer's disease that the value he gave to the practice of meditation was uppermost in his psyche. Meditation sustained him until his brain could no longer stay focused on the mantra. At age eighty, Edward 'retired' from the School; we spent half of the year in Florida. He soon realized how much he missed his participation in the School. With good friends Edward would speak rhapsodically about his School experiences. He began to show symptoms of Alzheimer's disease at age eighty-four. As the illness progressed, Edward suffered bouts of depression. At times he would tell me how lost he felt because he no longer received the fine energy the School offered. I would tell him that he still had the Teaching in his heart. He would respond, with a rueful smile, "yes, and the sannyasin retires to the forest to conclude his spiritual quest. But could I even find the forest now?"

Introduction

On an evening in December 2022, in his fifth year of experiencing the degenerative effects of Alzheimer's disease and four months before his death, my husband, Edward, was sitting in the living room with his family. He was eighty-eight years old. His two sons, John and James, with their wives and two teenage boys each, had gathered to welcome Edward's niece, Christina. She and her husband, Donald, had driven from Pittsburgh to be with her favorite uncle. The Christmas tree lights were lit; a fire was dancing in the wood stove. It was a festive time of year, and we were enjoying this evening of family unity. Edward was dozing off, his listless body slumped in the wing-back chair. Suddenly he lifted his body to an erect position, made eye contact with people in the room and began quietly, but with confidence, to conduct a class in philosophy. For forty-three years he had been a student and tutor at The School of Practical Philosophy where the study of Advaita Vedanta had been our life's work and Edward's devotional center. Advaita Vedanta is the study of the one unitary consciousness that envelops and characterizes the whole universe. [1]

As he began to speak the room fell quiet, as if everyone was holding their breath. We were in awe of the melodious voice, the inner stillness Edward displayed, and the exactitude of the Socratic method of question and response which he elicited from his listeners. I don't remember the whole sequence of the twenty-minute class, but no one moved a muscle. When he would ask something – for example, "are you watching the mind?... Do you feel the stillness behind the movements of mind?... Isn't this what we are?... Are you present right now?... *Now*?" – he would wait patiently for a response with full presence of mind. His main partner in the verbal exchange was his niece's husband, Donald, who sat next to him. Donald was intrigued by the conversation. Though a religious man, he had never encountered this probing type of entry into the realm of spirit. Edward was not only displaying normalcy. He was also offering a burst of brilliance and lucidity that was penetrating each of us as we listened. Despite the illness, the ability to reason and speak cogently about the teaching he loved was fully functioning for those twenty minutes. That this was possible was due to the presence of awareness, or consciousness, which underlies the functions of the mind and its physical instrument, the brain.

What you will read in the following chapters is a science-based, spiritual inquiry into Alzheimer's disease. The book's objective is twofold. It is an account of the six-year journey that my husband and I took through the progressive stages of Alzheimer's disease. That account relies upon daily journal entries that I kept over the years as his sole caregiver. It is also an argument in support of the proposition that the person living with Alzheimer's is, first, a person, not an entity with the unfortunate fate of being trapped in the prison of a deteriorating brain. This personhood is eloquently and forcefully argued in John Zeisel's book *I'm Still Here*. But more importantly, it will be proposed that the person is in essence a spiritual being, an embodied *soul*. The soul within the body remains untouched by the affliction that the body is experiencing. This spiritual essence is sometimes referred to as consciousness or awareness. It is also referred to as Mind in its largest sense. Even as the person living with Alzheimer's and the caregiver witness the alarming loss of normal neurological processes, the subtle embodied awareness is not affected. Awareness is not dependent upon the brain nor affected by its degenerative condition. In other words, it is argued that this essential awareness is a spiritual trait, embodied in human beings, that persists even in mental disorders that destroy parts of the brain. Jesus says, "the Kingdom of God is within you."[2] In the *Bhagavad Gita*, the god-man Krishna instructs Arjuna about the relationship of matter and spirit. Krishna says:

Thus in the body of man dwells the Supreme God.... Wherever life is seen in things movable or immovable, it is the joint product of Matter and Spirit.... As space, though present everywhere, remains by reason of its subtlety unaffected, so the Self, though present in all forms, retains its purity unalloyed.[3]

So, matter is infused with spirit, yet spirit is not bound by matter. The subtlety of spirit prevents us from locating it in matter which is what the empirical scientist in us is trained to do. The ability of Edward to conduct a class with heightened awareness even as his brain was deteriorating, suggests that one's identity is deeper than body, mind, or ego. The subtle energy of soul can pierce through the cognitive fog of Alzheimer's disease momentarily in the form of mental clarity and understanding, just as the sun's light can burst through clouds.

Throughout the book, there will be an effort to align a scientific understanding of Alzheimer's disease with this spiritual approach. Those interests which have been most important in life, those which feed the soul, are retained deep in the memory pockets of the brain, even the diseased brain. They are sustained long into the disease and even to the end of life. With the caregiver's help, these inner strengths and talents can be retrieved and amplified to nourish the soul and bring joy to the person living with Alzheimer's disease. Indeed, it is an interesting fact that the amygdala, a major structure in the brain for the retention of emotional memory and intelligence, has a prominent role throughout life. Early in human evolution, the amygdala is tasked with detecting predators through the fight-or-flight reflex. Its healthy functioning remains until late in the progression of Alzheimer's disease. Emotional sensitivity, active within the person living with Alzheimer's, acts as a thermometer of the emotional energies of people around him or her. Edward remained sensitive to these subtle energies in other people long into the disease. Positive emotional responses, like empathy for self and others, can be encouraged in the person living with Alzheimer's disease. When activities are introduced that bring pleasure and satisfaction, a feeling of happiness can, for a time, dispel negative emotions like depression. It remains a question as to whether awareness – the bedrock of the soul's existence – diminishes as brain tissue decays. In the hours preceding death, when the person is bedridden and cannot speak, it is hard for the observer to know whether awareness is still present, but if it is, then awareness guides the soul into the transition that death signals.

As caregiver, one needs to understand what is going on in the brain as the disease of Alzheimer's progresses. A rudimentary knowledge of brain science (neuroscience) allows for objectivity in dealing with eruptions of anger and personal insult directed at the caregiver by the person living with Alzheimer's disease. This scientific knowledge is married to an allegiance to spiritual truths that can fortify the caregiver emotionally. The most important duty of the caregiver is to remember the underlying, though invisible and ineffable, spiritual essence of the afflicted person. This will help the caregiver deal effectively and compassionately with times of inner frustration, impatience, and total lack of confidence in the ability to do the job that has been thrust upon her. It will also remind her to remind the beloved she serves of who he really is. This truth can be spoken, as in 'I am not this body, this mind, nor this ego: I am the Self – pure, conscious and blissful.'[4]

This task of reinforcing memory is aided by the breakthrough discovery in neuroscience of neuroplasticity. This is the capacity of the brain to restructure itself, to rebuild and rewire. There are two types of neuroplasticity: experience-dependent and self-directed. In the former, experiences are received and stored unconsciously in the basal ganglia of the brain, resulting in habitual acts that may or may not be beneficial. A glass of wine before dinner may bring pleasure, triggering a shot of dopamine. But the danger of becoming an alcoholic is also a possibility. Self-directed neuroplasticity is intentional. There is a conscious choice made in the prefrontal cortex, which is the command center of our uniquely human brain. If I decide to eat more nutritious food, and I notice my health and energy increasing, I will continue to eat healthfully. My brain is being rewired to continue the beneficial dietary change.

In the early stage of Alzheimer's, and even as the disease progresses, positive experiences will stimulate the neural circuits of the brain in advantageous ways. Meditation, mindful walking in the natural world, recounting of good memories, enjoying pleasures as simple as a leisurely meal with friends, tapping dormant talents like painting or playing a musical instrument, going to the theatre or a concert – all these activities can bring rest, zest, and happiness to the person living with Alzheimer's disease. Neuropsychologist Rick Hanson calls the repeated internalizing of positive experiences "taking in the good." [5] Hanson explains that, early in human evolution, a negativity bias developed in the brain to meet threats in the natural environment. The ability to react rapidly to a predator was a means to protect self and kin. *Taking in the good* depresses this negativity bias. Researchers at the Swiss Federal Institute of Technology in Zurich (ETH Zurich) conducted a recent study in which 261 participants split into two groups. One group meditated daily for fifteen minutes. The other group listened to calming music. It was found that those who meditated were objective about negative information presented to them. They were less controlled by negative emotions and therefore better able to make wise decisions in response. [6]

Taking in the good allows the soul to emerge and guide the life of the person living with Alzheimer's disease. As an example of self-directed neuroplasticity, *taking in the good* raises an enticing question: is it possible that Alzheimer's disease might be slowed down and even reversed if, through meditative practices, the mind directs the brain to repair and rebuild itself? In this healing work, the neurons infected with toxic proteins would be transmuted into healthy nerve cells. Although this idea may seem radical, averse to empirical study and verification, it will inform our exploration of the mind-body continuum in the second chapter entitled *Brain, Mind and Consciousness.* [7]

14

Meditation has been shown to reduce chronic pain, anxiety, and high blood pressure which can trigger heart attacks, strokes, and other ailments. Areas of the brain involved in attention, learning, memory, and mood regulation are strengthened through meditation. In September of 2019, researchers witnessed Tibetan Buddhist monks demonstrate the power of meditation. The monks covered their bodies with soaking wet sheets, sat in a very cold room, and meditated for an hour. They were able to change their metabolism, creating bodily heat. At the end of the hour the sheets were dry.

To summarize, it is proposed that there is an embodied awareness – a soul or spiritual essence – that resides in the body. This essence shines through the mind and the mind's physical manifestation: the brain. Though the soul resides in the body, it also transcends the limits of the body. It persists undisturbed and can be nourished in the person living with Alzheimer's disease, despite the progressive degeneration of brain tissue. For example, there is potent spiritual energy that is released when the caregiver offers loving words from the heart to the person living with Alzheimer's disease. In that moment of true empathy, the imagined gap between 'me' and 'you' disappears; the two souls meet. It helps if both the person living with Alzheimer's and his caregiver are already spiritually attuned through meditative practices accrued over a major portion of their lives. But it is never too late to begin a mindful, meditative approach to life. The late Thich Nhat Hanh, Buddhist teacher and advocate of mindfulness, reminds us that:

We can touch the Kingdom of God in everyday life. There is no need to travel a great distance to touch the

Kingdom of God, because it is not located in space or time. The Kingdom of God is in your heart. It is in every cell of your physical body. With a single mindful breath, a single insight that is deep enough, you can touch the Kingdom of God.[8]

Daily life is the schoolroom where both the person living with Alzheimer's disease and his caregiver can discover the Kingdom of God that dwells in the heart. Through their joint efforts in being mindful, healing energy circulates in their minds and bodies. As Jesus said: "When two or more are gathered in my name there am I in the midst of them." [9]

A perfect tableau for transformation.

Chapter One: **First Signs**

In 2019, as our story begins, we are living in Gardiner, N.Y. at the base of the Shawangunk mountains in the Hudson Valley. 2019 is the first year in which Alzheimer's disease is diagnosed in Edward, but symptoms go back to 2018. The appearance of odd behavior in people with Alzheimer's, even decades before diagnosis, is common. The following chronicle of first signs is taken from a journal I kept throughout the six years of Edward's journey through Alzheimer's disease.

For the latter six months of 2018, I noticed in Edward some anomalous behavior such as putting dishes away in the wrong places, but because he had always had some difficulty with kitchen clean-up duty it did not seem unusual. When he put an empty sour cream container in the fridge, peanut butter in the freezer, and left a half can of wet cat food in a cabinet, I became concerned. This misplacement of objects would continue and worsen throughout the six years in which my husband lived with the symptoms of Alzheimer's disease. One day, I saw that he was not wearing his wedding ring, nor the necklace with the single pearl that I had given him. "I don't know where they are," he said, "maybe I took them off when we went swimming." They were never found.

He began to forget conversations soon after they occurred, repeated questions like "how old am I?", "do we live here?", or "where do I sleep?" He didn't appear to hear my responses, so the dialogue became repetitive and disconnected. His need for me to repeat sentences seemed to show not only cognitive impairment but also hearing loss. I persuaded him to have his hearing checked. Hearing aids were prescribed but he refused to wear them. I noticed that, with friends and family, he began to have trouble following and understanding conversations. He couldn't keep up with the pace. He got confused, and, if he did speak, would remark on a topic which had already been discussed. That he was aware of this deficit was evident in his tendency to keep quiet and thus not be embarrassed. He couldn't remember the ordinary ways of doing things like washing dishes with soap; he would only rinse them. Sometimes he appeared oblivious of these unusual behaviors. Short-term memory loss is a typical sign of the onset of Alzheimer's disease. As the disease progressed and connections between the prefrontal cortex and other regions of the brain – especially the temporal and parietal lobes – atrophied, he put dishes away with food still on them.

After Thanksgiving, we went to Florida to stay at our Dunedin condo for five months. I noticed that Edward became moody. He would get depressed – a deviation from his usual even temperament. He continued to misplace things and have trouble following logical sequences of thought and expression, but now he would get frustrated with these behaviors. He ascribed them to aging; but he was a young eighty-four: trim and limber. Paying bills and doing the taxes became difficult. He became ultra-sensitive to what he perceived as slights or criticism. We got into more arguments. When I asked him to make a lectern for me, since I was scheduled to teach a class at Eckerd College in St. Petersburg, he consented but found the work challenging. He was using some pieces of wood stored in the garage. He had arranged his tools neatly on a pegboard. As an expert cabinetmaker this task would have been an easy one, but he fumbled, taking four days to complete the job instead of one day. Edward recognized that something was wrong but blamed his ineptitude on the materials. His confusion in understanding and executing measurements of the drawing I gave him would not have happened several years ago. Another sign of a growing inability to do basic carpentry work was the installation of a cabinet he had built up north and brought down to put in our condo kitchen. I noticed the bottom edge of the cabinet was rough and the hardware unevenly placed.

Around Christmas time, we found out that his brother Ludge (Polish for *Walter*) had been diagnosed with Alzheimer's disease. Ludge had become confused and forgetful. After he wrecked his car, Christina, his niece, persuaded him to be tested for dementia. She began caring for him as he was a widower; his wife, Helen, had died five years earlier. I began to suspect that Edward might have Alzheimer's disease also, but I didn't know how to approach the possibility with him. If he did have the disease, was it hereditary? Could it be a genetic flaw?

February – March 2019

In February 2019, Edward turned eighty-five. He slept longer in the mornings. It was harder to get him up for meditation which we had been practicing together twice a day for forty years. In March, Edward began taking a Japanese brush painting class at the Dunedin Art Center. This activity perked him up and he was avid in his daily practice

On the next page is one of his paintings.

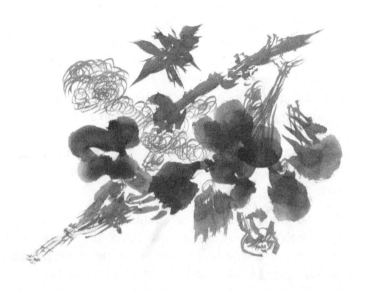

Image 2: Japanese brush painting by Edward

Edward consented to a verbal test for dementia from our doctor in Florida. He missed a few responses on math; he didn't know the day's date or the name of the president of the United States. He was given a set of three words which he would need to repeat to the doctor later in the interview. He only remembered one of them. The doctor, with my prompting, said that a more determinate diagnosis required a PET scan. The insurance company wouldn't pay for the procedure unless we first had a CAT scan of the brain. We had the CAT scan done. It showed normal deterioration of nerve cells due to aging. Edward used this result to resist a further PET scan. Perhaps he feared the results. I convinced him that certainty was necessary. He continued to resist; we argued. I kept saying that, for both our sakes (as I would be his caregiver), we needed to know the facts. Eventually he complied, still insisting that his brain activity was normal. He was just getting old.

On April 25th, he was given the PET scan. It showed deterioration of the temporal and parietal lobes. These areas had not absorbed the sugar dilution that the PET scan procedure administers – a first sign of neural degeneration. In reviewing the scan his doctor informed us that the results were indicative of Alzheimer's disease. He recommended two medications. Edward would start with Namenda (Memantine). After three months, he would add Aricept to his regimen.[10] Edward's brother was on Aricept only. We were told that these medications can slow down the inevitable progress of the disease by a year or so. Given in sequence, they are supposed to restore some of the connectivity between nerve endings at synapses in the brain. In Alzheimer's disease these connections are compromised. As it turned out, he stayed on Memantine for three years but discontinued Aricept after two days because it had a psychotic effect on him. I started reading *The 36-Hour Day* by Nancy L. Mace and Peter V. Rabins. Published in 1981, it was the first book devoted to Alzheimer's disease and other dementias.

Alzheimer's disease is a type of dementia. Dementia is a syndrome. About 80 per cent of dementia cases are Alzheimer's. Its symptoms are not present in normal aging. The disease was first discovered and described by Alois Alzheimer, a German neuropathologist, in 1906. In 1980, the non-profit health organization, Alzheimer's Association, was founded to advance the care and support of people with the disease. AA also provides research opportunities to better understand the disease and available treatments. According to the Centers for Disease Control and the National Institute of Aging, the number of people diagnosed with Alzheimer's disease is growing, in tandem with a growing global population. The increase in cases cannot simply be attributed to the fact that people live longer. Both the CDC and the NIA cite risk factors such as high body mass (obesity) and high blood sugar (diabetes) – neither of which Edward had. Perhaps two other risks, which we all face, should be added to these two factors: environmental pollution and the corrosive effect of stress on the mind-body from the constant incursions of our fast-paced, technologically advanced culture.

Alzheimer's disease is the seventh leading cause of death in the United States. More than six million Americans, aged sixty-five and older, are living with Alzheimer's disease. Globally, the estimate of people diagnosed with Alzheimer's is forty-four million, a number which could triple by 2050. Because Alzheimer's disease is terminal and progresses slowly, the physical and psychological burden of its effects falls not only on the person living with the disease but also on the caregiver and the person's family. It is in this context that I have learned two lessons that might benefit others dealing with the disease:

1) the necessity of an educated, science-based understanding of the disease by the afflicted person (although denial may prevent this), the caregiver, and family members; and

2) consideration by all parties of an approach to treatment that recognizes the spiritual integrity of the person living with Alzheimer's disease. This recognition is important because, as the brain tissue deteriorates, it is tempting to equate that loss with the loss of the person's humanity.

Although there is a common progression in Alzheimer's disease, it does not uniformly present itself. In her book *Spectrum of Hope*, neurologist Dr. Gayatri Devi explains that people may experience the disease in different ways. Influential factors could include personality, temperament, life experiences, and the availability of a good support group. According to a 2008 study of the prefrontal cortex, published in the *Indian Journal of Psychiatry*, patients with Alzheimer's disease who have a higher education and a skilled occupation have a neuropsychological advantage in that these accomplishments play a protective role in slowing down cognitive deterioration.[11] A daily meditation practice, which Edward followed for more than fifty years, has been shown to serve as a stimulant to the health of the brain. In fact, studies show that mindfulness training – the basis of meditation – stimulates the prefrontal cortex which is the latest evolutionary development in the human brain. When one adds simple physical exercises, such as a daily walk, mind-body health is sustained, and this rejuvenation can help to slow the progression of the disease. Sudden changes, like a move to a new house or frequent vacations, can have a negative impact, accelerating symptoms. I learned about this impact the hard way.

April – July 2019

As the art classes continued, Edward's artistic flair was on display; the experience nourished his self-confidence. Edward told me that the teacher would often ask him to lead a meditation at the beginning of the class to quiet the participants and allow the creative impulse to arise. This privilege was right in his wheelhouse. He was asked to present one of his paintings at the Center's art show at the end of the course.

23

Coming back to New York in late April, Edward seemed to hold steady but complained of being in a 'funk'. Adjusting to changes in location is hard for people with Alzheimer's. The efficiency of the processes of perception and memory in the new environment is tested. Fatigue sets in. At the time, I did not appreciate this fact. Reflecting now, it is obvious that even without the disease the demands of a vacation in a new place can be taxing. On vacation, we experience a heightened sense of presence, taking in every image, savoring every new site. We easily absorb and remember the activities of each day. Time slows down because of each day's richness. Those living with Alzheimer's disease cannot count on the brain to register, enjoy, and remember this rapid sequence of new sights and activities. Returning home is an abrupt transition and can be disorienting.

Another change in venue happened in June with a guided river cruise up the Danube. We had booked the trip a year ago. The tight schedule of walking tours and the busy agenda exhausted Edward. He was able to join conversations with fellow travelers by being quiet most of the time. Sometimes he came out with a quirky remark that made our new acquaintances laugh. I encouraged him to try to participate more; he made an acceptable effort. Our new friends couldn't know him as he used to be, gregarious and even intense when engaged in conversations about the teaching of Advaita or the theatre. In the past he would recite reams of Shakespeare soliloquies and sonnets and awe his audience with dramatic renditions of Keats's poems. In fact, that ability to remember these well-rehearsed lines remained until he reached an advanced stage of the disease.

In Prague, our last stop of the cruise, the weather turned very hot. Edward announced that we hadn't been out at all that day because of the heat. We had been out, twice.

That evening, at dinner, I said, "We're going to a Vivaldi concert."

Then, after dinner, he asked, "When is the movie? What is it?"

"It's not a movie," I said, "it's a concert."

This mismatched dialogue happened two more times before we left the restaurant.

The next morning, he woke up late. There was a city tour planned for our group. He said he didn't want to go. I told him to take the key card to our room and go down to the hotel dining room to have breakfast and that I would be back at 1:00. When I returned to the hotel room, he was sitting on a chair, looking confused and sullen. He said that he had had coffee in the room but never left the room to have breakfast. He didn't remember where I was or where to go for his morning meal. I was shocked and I said (which I should not have said) "it's Alzheimer's." He reacted angrily.

"We have to face this," I said, "call it what it is. We have the Teaching to remind us of who we are. 'You are not Alzheimer's disease. You are the Self.'"

He didn't respond. I was thinking, is this the beginning of my not being able to leave him without risking this forlorn and confused reaction which he called "feeling discombobulated"? I realized that the cruise was an overload on his brain.

Returning home on July 2nd, Edward slept a lot and was disoriented. The feeling of being disoriented and fatigued is more apt to occur and increase around dusk. This recurring emotional state is called *the sundown syndrome*. To some extent, fatigue is a natural experience for all of us at the end of a busy day. Fatigue relates to the normal biological clock – night owls excepted – but in Alzheimer's disease, fatigue spreads into the day as the disease progresses. This is understandable, as the brain is increasingly handicapped.

On July 5th, after meditation, Edward wanted to talk.

"We shouldn't have gone on the cruise," he said.

I sensed that his discomfort was related to his being unable to 'perform' with other people. He was aware that his brain could not function normally and he feared the inevitable progress of Alzheimer's disease, but didn't want to admit it. Denial was a safer course.

"I feel lost," he said. "I feel I am a burden to you." But then he followed that statement with: "I feel pressure from you because I'm decrepit."

This defensive move was upsetting. The words we exchanged were not without bitterness, resentment, and anger. After this exchange he sat glum and stone-faced. I realized there was a profound change happening in the power dynamic of our relationship. He was less emotionally in control of himself, and he felt weak. Is Alzheimer's worse for men who are conditioned in Western culture to be strong, reasonable, and steady? This cultural conditioning may persist despite the men's movement in sensitivity training that rose on the heels of feminism in the 1990s with Robert Bly's workshops.

After a period of silence, I said to him, "You are not decrepit; your body has an illness; we can look at this together, accept it, change our minds about it." He just looked at me.

As I said these words I thought, how would I feel if I knew I was losing my mind? I will be taking on more responsibilities now. I needed to accept this new job as caregiver without making him feel useless. I told myself to accept the situation. I needed to use humor, patience, and kindness without condescension, to pull him out of moodiness, out of depression. Could I do this? Alzheimer's disease has a particularly potent negative connotation. It projects a cultural stigma that presents the afflicted person as weak and feeble-minded. It will be my job to remind us both of what we believe: that each person's higher self is the *Atman* which is *Brahman*, or God, in embodied form. *Atman* is forever pure, conscious, and blissful. *Tatvamasi, I am That*.

How the Human Brain Works

As the reality of being my husband's primary caregiver sank in, I knew I had to learn more about the human brain and nervous system, and how the breakdown of their normal functioning takes place. In this section, the facts of neural physiology are examined. These facts assume normal cognitive and emotional behavior. A contrast will then be drawn between normal brain functioning and the abnormal neurological signs revealed in Edward's words and actions as Alzheimer's disease takes hold.

The human brain consists of eighty-six billion nerve cells. It is bilateral in structure, having a right and left hemisphere. Connecting the two hemispheres is the corpus callosum – a thick, flat bundle of nerve cells under the cerebral cortex that facilitates communication between the hemispheres. There are specific functions delegated to each hemisphere. For example, the right hemisphere processes holistic visual-spatial information while the left hemisphere processes language abilities such as speech production and comprehension. Each hemisphere contains the four lobes of the cerebrum – frontal, parietal, temporal, and occipital. Each lobe plays a role in the brain's operation. Structures with specific functions reside in each lobe and, because there are two hemispheres, there are two of each structure. For example, memory storage happens in the two hippocampi that sit on the underside of the temporal lobes. Below is a diagram of the left hemisphere of the brain. The four lobes are labeled, along with additional structures which will be dealt with later.

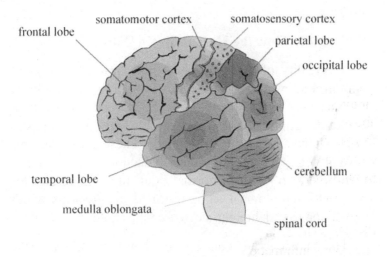

Image 3: Four lobes of the cerebrum *courtesy of*
www.wikipedia.org

Although the four lobes fulfill specific functions, they do not exist in isolation from each other. Just as the body is an interconnected whole of individual parts, so the structures of the brain communicate with each other. The cerebrum, or cerebral cortex, is also called the neocortex because 90 per cent of it is evolutionarily newer in human development. The four lobes carry out many operations including executive functions such as attention, memory, language, and planning as well as motor and sensory activation and control.

To effectively execute its many functions, the brain is constructed in folding layers. There are six layers of outer gray matter in the cerebral cortex; the inner area of the brain is white matter. These folds are like the hills and valleys of a landscape. The hills are called gyri, the valleys sulci. The supramarginal gyrus, for example, is in the parietal lobe. It participates in working memory tasks such as mathematical calculation in the left hemisphere. In the right hemisphere, this gyrus has an important role in visuospatial awareness and feeling empathy for others. The central sulcus stretches horizontally across the skull, separating two bands of gray matter – the sensory and motor cortices. These bands are labeled in the diagram above. The lateral sulcus separates the temporal from the frontal and parietal lobes. Deep underneath the cerebral cortex are the basal ganglia. These clusters of neurons provide feedback to the cortex regarding learning. They also assist in fine-tuning and executing movements. Damage to these neurons is associated with Parkinson's disease. The basal ganglia are also a meeting point where emotional information connects to the motor circuitry to influence action. For example, feeling empathy for someone may elicit a hug.

There are two nervous systems in the human body. The central nervous system comprises the brain and the spinal cord. This is the command center. The peripheral nervous system comprises the sensory and motor neuron networks throughout the body that carry messages to and from central command. If you stub your toe, for example, the sensory nerves in your toe immediately send a signal by means of the peripheral nervous system up through the spinal cord and thalamus to the cerebral cortex. The stimulus takes one hundredth of a second to reach the brain which then signals the motor neurons to assuage the pain. Your fingers begin to massage your toe. The efficacy of this messaging system is due in large part to the myelin sheath made of protein and fatty substances which surrounds and insulates nerve cells. Damage to the myelin slows down communication between cells.

The autonomic nervous system is a further breakdown of the peripheral nervous system. As its name suggests, the nerve cells behave automatically. They are separated into two divisions – the parasympathetic and the sympathetic. The parasympathetic division is responsible for involuntary movements such as breathing, heartbeat, and body temperature. Fortunately, we do not have to consciously regulate these functions. For example, we are usually not even aware of the breath, unless we are on a hike up a steep mountain, aware of our breathlessness, or practicing a type of meditation like mindful breathing. The parasympathetic division has been labeled as the 'rest and digest' state of the body.

The sympathetic division of the autonomic nervous system is controlled by the hypothalamus and works together with its complement, the parasympathetic division. The sympathetic division is summoned into action by emergency situations such as a stressful event. When something is perceived and felt as a threat, the fight-or-flight reaction is triggered. Common examples are feeling very nervous right before a performance or jumping back with a gasp when a rope on the road is perceived as a snake. The amygdala immediately goes into action. It sends a distress signal via the neural network in the brain to the hypothalamus which then activates the sympathetic nervous system by sending signals to the pituitary gland which in turn sends a message to the adrenal glands to pump the neurotransmitter adrenaline into the bloodstream. Physical signs of this autonomic reaction are immediate: blood pressure rises, hands get clammy, heart beats faster, skin flushes or pales, bladder may release urine, the liver, glucose – all this in a few seconds at most and at some cost since the equilibrium of the resting state (the parasympathetic system) has been breached in response to danger. The efficiency of this reaction has been honed over the centuries, tracing back to the need in our evolutionary history to be on the lookout for predators like bears or lions. Today we face predators of our own making like global warming and a fast-paced, media-rich culture that invites hypertension and other health risks. Practices that calm the nerves, like seated or walking meditation, are valuable antidotes to the stresses of our time, for the healthy individual as well as the person living with Alzheimer's disease.

The Four Lobes

By examining the functions of the four lobes of the brain and their internal structures we can contrast healthy functioning of the brain with the abnormal effects of

Alzheimer's disease. The four lobes often integrate their specific information and overlap in their functioning despite the sulci that separate them. The fact that the brain works holistically is both a plus and a minus for persons living with Alzheimer's: a plus because built-in redundancy and compensation for damaged areas can sometimes counteract the progression of Alzheimer's disease; a minus because damaged nerve cells in the brain and spinal cord do not as a rule regenerate and their decay leads to neurodegeneration.

The frontal lobe

The frontal lobe is the largest of the four lobes. It initiates mental and physical actions. Mediated by the neurotransmitter dopamine, the frontal lobe integrates information sent from various areas of the brain, such as the sensory reception areas, and puts into action executive functions such as attention, motivation, abstract thinking and comprehension, planning and decision-making, discernment, impulse control, memory, and learning. Physically it initiates and coordinates voluntary movements through the pre-motor and primary motor cortices, including voluntary muscles of the eyes, face, and limbs. It also controls the muscles for the articulation and production of speech.

The most recent evolutionary development in the frontal lobe is the pre-frontal cortex (PFC) which takes up one third of the cerebral cortex. The PFC mediates cognitive and emotional aspects of the personality. It acts as an overseer of the other regions of the brain, regulating thoughts, actions, and emotions. The PFC regulates the executive functions mentioned above, as well as being the site of self-awareness and creativity. Awareness as working memory is in the upper outer portions of the PFC in contrast to lower middle areas where social-emotional content is processed. The PFC regulates emotions through wide neural connections with other regions of the brain, such as the limbic system which is comprised of structures in the temporal lobes.

The anterior cingulate cortex (including the cingulate gyrus), abbreviated as ACC, sits below the pre-frontal cortex. The PFC and the ACC work together to integrate thinking and feeling. The ACC joins logical reasoning with emotional intelligence. Studies have found that meditation, one function of which is to integrate the mind and heart in positive ways, strengthens the ACC. The ACC helps in the focusing of attention, transforming intention into action through working memory. Edward's woodworking profession was successful because of his focused attention, extraordinary skill, and precision of movement. When he contracted Alzheimer's disease, his ability to work gradually eroded, especially in the sequencing of tasks and the memory of how that sequencing is ordered so that the intended goal – the finished product – is envisioned. Did the degeneration of the interface between the PFC, the ACC, and structures in the temporal lobes contribute to this loss of a fundamental part of Edward's persona? The knowledge that he was losing these abilities caused him to withdraw. He would use some excuse not to do simple tasks, revealing that he was aware of the loss. The outbursts of frustration and anger that would arise in the later stages of the disease, when he couldn't do something as simple as putting on his clothes correctly, indicate damage to the PFC. Two of the PFC's roles – the organizing of sequential actions and the restraining of negative emotions – were compromised. We all have moments of frustration and anger, but we have the choice to inject reason over emotion and thereby restore mental balance. This choice diminishes as lesions appear in the brain tissue of the frontal lobe.

The ACC has strong connections with the anterior insula which is located deep within the lateral sulcus that separates the temporal, parietal, and frontal lobes. The anterior insula is like a crossroad. It senses the changing states of the body, as sensations and feelings are relayed to it by the brainstem, spinal cord, and thalamus. It picks up these subjective feeling states – our gut feelings (there are neurons even in the digestive system!) – and relays them to the limbic regions. The anterior insula is also involved in the processing of this cognitive and emotional information in cortical areas of regulation and integration like the PFC and ACC. Pathologies that reveal abnormal subjective feelings such as generalized anxiety, depression, and mood disorders are characteristic of dementia. In Alzheimer's disease, these pathologies are joined by a loss of the sense of self due to a decrease in gray matter in the insula, causing dysfunctionality.[12] As the disease progressed, Edward often relied on items like his wallet, cell phone, or watch to assure him of his identity. When he forgot where he had placed these items, he became anxious. Depression also increased, particularly a feeling of uselessness. One cannot help but speculate about whether deficits in the insula were involved.

The above description of the integrative communication between the PFC, ACC, and anterior insula demonstrates the complexity and refined neural connections between areas of the brain. It reveals the brain's holistic structure and functioning.

The parietal lobe

The central sulcus, and its adjacent primary motor and

somatosensory cortex bands on either side, separate the frontal lobe from the parietal lobe. The somatosensory cortex on the side of the parietal lobe registers and processes sensory information. This information is conveyed to it by sensory neurons in the body's peripheral nervous system which pick up information from the sense organs. The parietal lobe recognizes, analyzes, and remembers sensations like touch, pain, temperature, pressure, vibrations, and awareness of spatial relationships. Sensing where one's body is in space and recognizing the body's surroundings is called *proprioception*. These tasks require knitting together visual, auditory, and somatosensory stimuli as they arise from the spinal cord, travel up to the cerebellum, and then to the parietal lobe. The posterior section of the sensory association cortex, which is a large area that includes the supramarginal gyrus, dips into both occipital (visual) and temporal lobes. This section is where proprioception is most active. If, for example, one rises from a chair and, through a decision in the PFC, intends to walk across the room, sensory neurons are alerted, and axons of motor neurons are immediately directed from the cerebral cortex to the muscles in the legs. One begins to walk. Disruption of this mostly unconscious exchange can result in the loss of proprioception. The brain loses touch with the body and its immediate environment. The cerebellum can also be involved because it coordinates bodily movements, making them smooth and efficient. Lesions in the cerebellum can create jerky body movements. Coordinated movement becomes sporadic at best.

In his book *The Man Who Mistook His Wife for a Hat,* neurologist Oliver Sacks describes a patient, Christina, who had no sense of her body in space. Her hands would wander, overshooting what she meant to pick up. She told

Dr. Sacks that she felt disembodied. She was finally diagnosed with a rare condition of sensory neuritis which affected the proprioceptive fibers in the sensory roots of spinal and cranial neurons. She was forced to depend upon her vision – her eyes – to orient her body in space to compensate for the loss of proprioception. As Alzheimer's disease progressed in Edward's body, his balance and ability to walk in measured steps became awkward. He would rise from the wing-back chair where he sat for hours during the day, stand unsteadily, and then, with my urging, begin to walk. After he had fallen three times in this effort, without injury, we began a routine of marching in place when he stood, to gain balance before walking. It was sad to see someone whose body could move with grace, both as a ballroom dancer and a master carpenter, lose that grace. Shortly before his death, after a fourth fall which was serious, he was bedridden and in some pain. He lost control of his arms which would flail in all directions. I held his hands to help him keep control over his arms.

It appears that the sensation of touch persists in awareness longer than the other senses. Hours before his death, Edward was aware of the touch we shared as my hand covered his. Our friend, Michael, whose wife Eileen had Alzheimer's disease for ten years, describes a time a few days before her death when she was bedridden and could no longer speak. They were lying side by side. Her eyes were closed; his hand was clasped in hers. He started to get up at one point and she grabbed his thumb. 'She knows,' he thought. And he said to her – as he had said many times before – "I know you're in there; you just can't get out."[13] Michael realized, just as I did, that awareness transcends the diseased brain.

The temporal lobe

On either side of the head, above and behind the ears, are the two temporal lobes. These, as well as the parietal lobes, show early damage in Alzheimer's disease. The temporal lobes contain structures that are important centers of memory (and thus learning), language production and comprehension, hearing (the primary and associated auditory cortices), and object recognition. New research shows specific regions in the temporal lobes for music perception and production (right lobe) and language perception and production (left lobe). Wilder Penfield (1891-1976), an American Canadian neurosurgeon, developed a procedure to cure epilepsy that involved stimulating areas of the temporal lobe that evoke memory. In an interesting experiment, in which he probed a certain region of the temporal lobe of a woman undergoing surgery, she reported that she heard a song played by instruments in a performance that she attended many years before. It was, she said, as if she were reliving that performance in the operating room.

Broca's area, which straddles the frontal and temporal lobes, is responsible for speech production. If this area is damaged, as in the advanced stages of Alzheimer's disease, aphasia, or loss of the ability to speak, can occur. Edward became progressively silent in the last month of his life. During the last days, he was unable to speak.

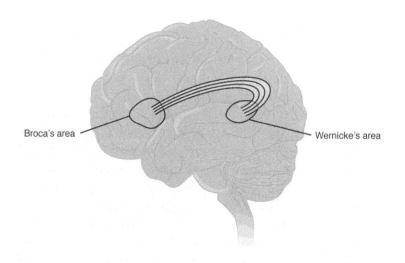

Broca's area

Wernicke's area

Image 4: Broca and Wernicke areas, *courtesy of*
www.commons.wikimedia.org

Wernicke's area spreads out between the primary auditory
area in the temporal lobe and visual areas of the parietal lobe
where sounds and visual stimuli are first processed.
Wernicke's area is focused on verbal understanding – what
we hear, digest, and comprehend. When there are lesions in
this region words might be articulated but they make no
sense. Edward's difficulty in keeping pace with and
understanding conversations was an early sign of temporal
lobe damage. In his last days, precipitated by a serious fall,
the Hospice nurse thought he might have had a stroke from
hitting his head on the metal baseboard against the wall.
When he tried to speak, sounds came out, but the words
were garbled and unintelligible.

Neuroscientists are finding that hearing loss makes a person more vulnerable to dementia. This relationship between hearing and brain health makes sense because hearing loss cuts off a major sensory tool that stimulates the mind-brain and connects a person to the world. The fact that Edward's hearing became impaired several years before he was diagnosed with Alzheimer's disease may have contributed to the progression of the disease, particularly as he rarely wore his hearing aids. Preventive measures, like keeping one's sensory faculties at optimum levels through regular eye and ear check-ups, are valuable in keeping the brain exercised and healthy, thus diminishing the risk of Alzheimer's.

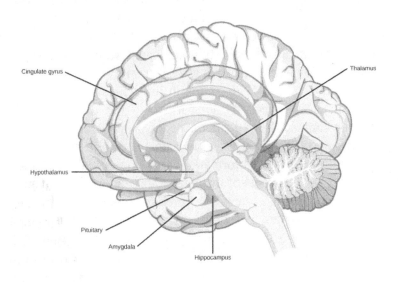

Image 5: The limbic system, courtesy of www.commons.wikimedia.org

The temporal lobe is a significant part of the limbic system – a group of structures that regulate memory and emotions. This lobe features three main structures of the limbic system: the amygdala, which is home to emotional arousal; the hippocampus, which encodes and stores memories; and the olfactory cortex, which is located deep inside the lobe. Smell affords object recognition. It is the oldest sense that we share with all animals. These internal structures of the temporal lobe are in proximity and work together, along with the thalamus and hypothalamus.

The amygdala is the site of feelings and emotions. It sits in the medial temporal lobe, just in front of the hippocampus. The PFC may assist in emotional arousal, especially in the case of subtle emotional responses, like generalized anxiety. As described earlier, the amygdala serves as an alarm bell. It is activated whenever one is feeling strong emotions such as fear or anger. The amygdala ignites the fight-or-flight reflex in the sympathetic nervous system. It is helped by its partners – the thalamus and hypothalamus. The thalamus, an egg-shaped structure in the center of the brain, serves as a relay station. It delivers sensory and motor information from the spinal cord and lower brain structures of the cerebellum and medulla to and from the cerebral cortex. The cerebral cortex of the frontal lobe then initiates a response to the situation through the cingulate cortex/gyrus, which drives the body to respond, either consciously or reflexively, to the emotions aroused, particularly those caused by pain or fear.

The hypothalamus is situated below and in front of the thalamus. The hypothalamus controls primal drives like hunger and sex. It regulates the endocrine system. In response to the alarm sent by the amygdala, the hypothalamus alerts the pituitary gland (which sits right below it) to release adrenaline. The hypothalamus also makes oxytocin which is stored in the back of the pituitary gland. This hormone is secreted when the skin is stimulated, as in sexual activity. This fact may be related to the importance of touch as a means of contact between the caregiver and the person who is living with Alzheimer's disease. Touch is the non-verbal signal of care, comfort, and safety. Neuroscientists have discovered that a subset of neurons in the mammillary body of the hypothalamus are subject to hyperactivity and degeneration. They are investigating whether the use of a drug that reverses the impairment of memory in epilepsy cases can treat these mammillary neurons in persons living with Alzheimer's disease.

Located right behind the amygdala, near the ear, is the hippocampus which is the main source of memory – both short-term and long-term memory. The latter is associated with learning from experience. The hippocampus is charged with storing memories, both positive and negative. Neural links exist between the amygdala and the hippocampus so that vivid memories, such as that of the woman in Penfield's experiment, can still evoke strong emotion. If the amygdala is receiving information that ignites feelings connected to an old trauma, it is the hippocampus that retains memories of that event as well as similar, linked traumatic experiences. Those memories are communicated to the amygdala to resolve the current traumatic situation. The hippocampus evaluates the situation and puts things in perspective. It controls how active the amygdala gets, and it can inhibit its expression. The PFC may get involved as well by inhibiting an emotional response, especially if it endangers the mind-body's health. The health of the American psyche was endangered because of the long-term emotional grief and anxiety prompted by the terrorist attack on the World Trade Center on 9/11/2001. Similarly, when Covid-19 struck in 2019 and became a long-term pandemic, the brain's emergency crew of amygdala, hippocampus, and PFC had to work overtime to stabilize the brain.

During the progression of Alzheimer's disease, Edward had less and less control over emotional outbursts as lesions spread in the brain tissue of the temporal lobe. When I suggested he do something like brush his teeth before bed he would often explode with remarks like "stop ordering me around!" Memories from married life in which he perceived that I was trying to control a situation would resurface, producing knee-jerk anger at the least provocation.

There are two types of memory: declarative, which is memory of facts and events, and procedural, which is memory of motor skills and routines. If the hippocampus has lesions, procedural memory is more likely to be retained for a longer time than declarative memory because the cerebellum helps to reinforce the learning and retaining of motor skills. Older, long-term memories of facts (declarative memory) are shown to be stable and lasting in many types of brain disease, including Alzheimer's. Even in the last month of his life, Edward remembered his birthplace in Pittsburgh, some of his friends that he grew up with, his brother, and especially his mother. But he couldn't remember the house where his mother lived or whether she was alive or dead. Edward often mistook his son, John, for his brother Ludge. In the early stage of the disease, when Edward got lost driving back home from the airport, he stopped several times at gas stations and once at a pub. He believed he was visiting friends from Pittsburgh and exhibited no fear or anxiety when he was finally found by the police.

Edward's short-term memory was affected even before diagnosis in 2019. The loss of recent memories continued for the next five years. For example, he would immediately forget what he had just said and what I had just said to him. He would forget that he just ate. In contrast, it was not until late in the progression of the disease that Edward found the motor skill of walking difficult. When this procedural memory faded his steps would be off balance and his muscular coordination compromised. Memory of more complex motor skills, such as those required for carpentry work, were affected early in the disease. Gaps in being able to perform a sequence of movements frustrated him.

The hippocampus has one other function, that of neurogenesis. It is the birthplace of new neurons. Neurogenesis may help to consolidate memory. It has been discovered that the new neurons produced by the hippocampus don't live very long and their production decreases with age. Still, it is believed by scientists that exercise, like walking, can stimulate their production. I encouraged Edward to walk outside with me every day. During the winter he would resist because of the cold, so sometimes we would just walk around the interior of the house. We designed a kind of indoor track that helped him remember where rooms were, and their functions, as we passed them.

Some cells in the hippocampus are *place cells*. They inform an animal (including us) of its spatial relationship to the environment. They help the animal recall previous places. Many animals use smell to detect places, humans not so much; but this would indicate a connection between the hippocampus and the olfactory cortex. New place cells appear when the environment changes to help with navigation. This adjustment would indicate an adaptive advantage. If the hippocampus undergoes damage, which is the case with Alzheimer's, then it is understandable that the person living with the disease would feel disoriented in new places. This disorientation was observed whenever Edward and I would go out – whether it was a shopping trip, a doctor's appointment, or a visit to one of our sons' houses where Edward had been many times. He often did not recognize where he was, and then, returning home, expressed feeling unfamiliar with his surroundings, until I pointed out something he could connect to, like the kitchen table. He would ask me, "Where are we? In Florida?"

"No," I would say, "New York. This is our home." There would be a brief period of anxiety, which I read in his face and voice, until he became grounded in the remembered sense of place.

Scientists are studying the possible connection between the hippocampus and the entorhinal cortex. The latter interfaces between the hippocampus, the cerebral cortex, and the parietal lobe. The entorhinal cortex mediates information going in and out of these areas. These connections show the holistic nature of the brain. They enable the coordination between memory, navigation, proprioception, and the perception of time. Edward often lost track of the day, date, time, and place.

The occipital lobe

The occipital lobe sits towards the back of the head. It

is the center for visual perception and analysis. The primary visual cortex makes us aware of visual stimuli. The adjacent visual association cortex processes this visual information so that we recognize and understand the meaning of what we see. Neural connections with the PFC necessarily allow for this understanding, especially if we are attentive in the moment. Attention is an executive function of the PFC. We remember what we see through neural connections to the hippocampus. If there is damage to the visual areas, several functions are compromised. In particular, the perception of depth, color, and movement are affected.

One day, when we were driving out of the parking lot at Lowe's, Edward suddenly shouted "stop!" I immediately put on the brakes, but then I saw that there was no obstacle in front of the car. He thought he saw a barrier that we were about to hit. The only 'barrier' was a Stop sign to our right. Sometimes, when he poured water into his teacup, he was not able to see when to stop pouring. The fact that Edward had macular degeneration may have compounded the visual damage occurring in the occipital lobe.

There are two neural pathways in the occipital lobe which can become damaged in Alzheimer's disease. In what is referred to as the *where* neural pathway, aspects of the visual image pass into and are shared with the parietal lobe where spatial location is ascertained. Damage to this pathway results in the inability to perceive distances. There is a second pathway, the *what* pathway, which connects the visual cortex to the inferior temporal cortex (IT) located at the base of the temporal lobe. The IT controls the recognition of objects, which in turn depends on memory. Thus, other structures like the hippocampus are involved.

When this pathway is impaired, objects are not readily identified. In the more advanced stages of Alzheimer's disease, Edward had difficulty recognizing the object he once knew as his wallet. He had trouble distinguishing the food on his dinner plate. He would 'see' broccoli and baked potato but not know what each vegetable was. "What is this?" he would ask.

Failure to recognize things is called *agnosia*. Oliver Sacks describes the case of Dr. P, a brilliant musician and teacher of music, who, despite a growing tumor in the visual parts of the brain, retained his musical talents until his death. However, he progressively lost the ability to recognize simple items like a pair of gloves that Dr. Sacks showed him. Dr. P. gave approximate measurements of the item and surmised the function of the inner space of the glove but could not name the item as a glove.

Prosopagnosia is the failure to recognize faces, even one's own face in the mirror. When I would mention a friend's name, Edward could not connect the name to the face. One day, an old friend appeared with a gift of hot soup and sandwiches for lunch. Edward didn't know who she was. It wasn't until late in the progression of the disease that Edward lost the ability to recognize some family members, including me. On the last day of his life, as he lay bedridden with his eyes closed and his daughter-in-law's hand in his, I came into the room and said something to her. Edward immediately reacted, his body stirring with excitement. Although he couldn't lift his head, or speak to acknowledge my presence, he knew I was there by the sound of my voice. The auditory cortex in the temporal lobe, and the pons, were still functional.

The Brainstem

In human evolution, the oldest and most basic part of the human brain is the brainstem. It is divided into three parts. The top part or mid-brain controls eye movements. Perhaps the permanent closing of the eyes at a normal death is a shutting down of this function. The middle part, the pons, coordinates hearing, facial movements, and balance. At the bottom of the brainstem is the medulla oblongata. It connects the spinal cord to the brain through ribbons of sensory (ascending) and motor (descending) axons. These axons facilitate the passage of information regarding bodily functions. The medulla plays an essential role in vital autonomic functions like breathing, heart rate, and swallowing. Inability to swallow is a sign that may appear in the late stage of Alzheimer's disease. It never occurred in Edward's case, but the instruction of the Hospice nurse shortly before Edward's death was that I shouldn't feed him. This instruction was based on both his lack of appetite but also the possibility he might choke if he couldn't swallow. Water is recommended in small doses and towards the end a moist swab wiped in and around the mouth.

In the underside of the medulla are groups of neurons called the reticular formation. They contain peptides and monoamines. Monoamine is a type of neurotransmitter that includes serotonin, adrenaline, and dopamine. The reticular formation affects the brain by its involvement in arousal and levels of consciousness or awareness. The thalamus – the relay station that sends signals from the brainstem to the higher cortices of the brain – is also involved with regulating levels of consciousness, like wakefulness and the sleep cycle. Lesions in the reticular formation can produce a loss of consciousness or stupor. Yet it can be argued that behind this catatonic state is awareness. There have been numerous cases of catatonia in which the body becomes frozen in space; the person is mute, unable to eat or drink. Often due to a motor or immune system disorder, these patients can be awakened, even after decades, sometimes by administering medication such as lorazepam. After awakening they describe the experience as feeling trapped in an inner world of fear and anxiety, but of full awareness.

Oliver Sacks worked in a clinic with patients who had post-encephalitic Parkinson's disease. His book *Awakenings* chronicles his work with these patients. Sacks believed that healing requires a humanistic, holistic approach that goes beyond the scope of neuroscience's brain-centered, mechanistic perspective. He saw each patient as a person and a spiritual being, suffering from a debilitating disease. Medication might help but just as important was the doctor's empathy and a nurturing environment. Included in the latter was rediscovering with the patient past experiences of joy that could, temporarily at least, bring them out of stupor and give them some quality of life. One Parkinsonian patient, Edith T., a former music teacher, complained that her movements had become wooden and that she couldn't dance anymore. She would periodically go into a frozen state that was both timeless and motionless. The only stimulants that brought her out of these episodes were contact, through touch, with another person, and music. Regarding the latter, she could describe, after awakening from stupor, how helpless she felt, until the music released her. She told Dr. Sacks that she needed to be *remusicked* to be revived.[14] Miss T's ability to speak of her experience of catatonia shows the existence of an underlying awareness in the mind-brain.

A Microscopic View of the Brain

What happens in the nerve cells of the brain to produce
Alzheimer's disease? Below is an image of a normal
neuron, showing the cell body, surrounded by dendrites.
The neuron has a long tail – an axon – that juts out from
the axon terminal.

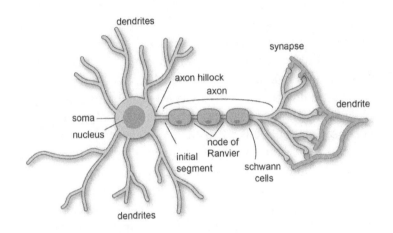

Image 6: Nerve cell, courtesy of www.wikimedia.org

An axon sends information from its neuron cell body to
another neuron that receives the information on the
dendrites of its cell body. The place of connection is called
a synapse. Cells communicate at synapses via the release
of an electrical or chemical signal. A simple analogy is
this: you order a medication from the drug store. A
messenger brings it to your door, rings the doorbell, you
answer the bell and receive the package. The messengers
that carry the signal from the dendrite via axon to the
neighbor neuron are neurotransmitters. These substances

bind to the dendrite at the receptor site, either stimulating or inhibiting activity in the receiving neuron. Maybe you don't answer the door thinking the visitor may be a thief! The neurons are supported by glial cells that serve as clean-up crew to remove cellular waste and/or toxic substances during transit.

In the Alzheimer brain, a progressive weakening and loss of neurons occurs due to the build-up and abnormal functioning of naturally occurring proteins called beta-amyloid and tau. The beta-amyloid proteins clump together, forming *plaque* at synapses. The plaque creates a barrier, thus obstructing neural connections. Tau proteins form neurofibrillary tangles in the cell body. A new research study at the University of Edinburgh discovered that these tangles, or tau oligomers, jump around at synapses and cut cells off from each other.[15] Normally, tau proteins help neurons stay healthy by attaching themselves to tiny tubules that guide nutrients from the cell to its dendrites and axon. In persons with Alzheimer's disease, tau proteins detach from these tubules and block the smooth transfer of stimuli to and from synapses by forming web-like tangles. One type of glial cells, called microglia, are unable to come to the rescue of the neurons to clear away the hazardous obstructions. Scientists don't know why their service is aborted. One hypothesis is the presence of a genetic abnormality in a gene called TREM2 which normally tells glial cells to remove plaque and thus reduce inflammation in the brain. A new imaging technique shows that another type of glial cells, called astrocytes, become infested with plaque; they also cannot perform clean-up duty. Moreover, they release chemicals that cause inflammation in the brain, attacking the neurons they are there to protect. This situation mimics autoimmune substances that attack their own cells. In experimenting with mice, neuroscientists at Stanford University have discovered that a certain drug, targeted at the kynurenine neural pathway that exists in both microglia cells and astrocytes, improved the brain's metabolism. As the drug cleared the pathway of beta-amyloid and tau proteins, the mice showed improved cognitive abilities and memory.[16]

Vascular problems may also be involved in the faulty functioning of neural connections in the brain due to Alzheimer's disease. For example, blood vessels in the brain fill with beta-amyloid plaques leading to mini-strokes. Thus, Alzheimer's disease is both a cause and an effect of vascular abnormalities. When Edward fell a few days before his death, the bodily response to the fall indicated the possibility of a stroke.

Neuroscientists are working to identify early stages of Alzheimer's disease through non-invasive means. If diagnosed at an early stage, the hope is that antidotes might be discovered that can stem neurodegeneration before it becomes irreversible. Research scientists at Cedars-Sinai Medical Center have discovered that the build-up of beta-amyloid proteins in the brain shows up in the blood vessels of the eyes. If diagnosed, this sign can provide early non-invasive detection of Alzheimer's disease.[17] There is also gut biome research which shows that there may be a parallel between an excessive accumulation of toxic beta-amyloid and tau proteins in the intestines and a similar build-up in the temporal and parietal lobes of the brain.[18] Studies are also showing a link between severe sleep apnea and an increased risk of dementia through build-up of plaque in memory areas like the hippocampus. The combination in Edward's health profile of hearing loss, macular degeneration, sleep apnea (though not severe it persisted for ten+ years), and a possible genetic component, may have made him risk prone.

The Stages of Alzheimer's Disease

The following is a brief sketch of the stages of Alzheimer's disease. Their boundaries are porous. Early signs, like short-term memory loss, continue and can worsen throughout the span of the disease. Each stage builds on the previous one, adding new impairments. Usually after diagnosis, a person with Alzheimer's disease lives for four to eight years but may live up to twenty years. The length of each stage varies from individual to individual. Edward's condition lasted for six years. In the two other case studies which are referenced, Eileen, Michael's wife, had Alzheimer's for ten years. Karen, David's wife, had Alzheimer's for four years after the diagnosis, but symptoms gradually became noticeable four years before the diagnosis. Timing depends upon how quickly the toxic proteins spread in the brain. A person living with Alzheimer's disease may die of some other cause before the brain tissue is fully destroyed.

- mild (early) stage: memory lapses, misplacing objects (even valuable ones); difficulty with familiar tasks at home or work, trouble organizing (e.g. paying bills); mild anxiety and agitation which heightens in the evening (sundown syndrome).

- middle (moderate) stage (the longest stage): confusion and difficulty in speaking and/or comprehending speech (e.g. following conversations); easily frustrated and angry (by the realization of reduced capacities); refusing to do routine acts like brushing the teeth or bathing (or saying he/she already did that but you know he/she didn't); changing sleep patterns; unable to match face with name of person he/she knows; confusion about where he/she is, disoriented (proprioception disrupted); repetitive questions (connected to memory loss), not knowing common facts like the day or date; increased tendency to get lost or wander; changes in personality (e.g. mood swings between confrontation and withdrawal); forgetting or getting confused about personal and family history.

- middle towards severe: delusionary, paranoid, and hallucinating behaviors; emotional outbursts (e.g. anger and suspicion aimed at caregiver) which can accompany persistent denial; difficulty choosing clothes or trouble putting them on; hygiene neglect; help needed for toileting and showering (shower chair and grab bars are helpful); less able to regulate bladder and bowels (use of Depends); mistaking friends and even family members for other people; sleeping more at night and dozing off during the day; loss of appetite.

- late (severe) stage: sleeping long hours, body less flexible; walking becomes difficult and even painful (walker may be necessary for balance as risk of falling rises indicating motor cortex damage); may need a hospital bed with adjacent commode; trouble lifting the head to sit up in bed; not wanting to eat; speaking less and eventually unable to speak; may lose ability to swallow; requires twenty-four hour care as he/she becomes bedridden. The most common cause of death is pneumonia. A severe fall may also precipitate a terminal state. The services of Hospice can be called in at the late stage, usually around six months before death. This allows the loved one to die at home. The Hospice nurses are trained to know the signs of impending death. Their attentive care is empathetic and skilled both for the person living and dying with Alzheimer's disease and the caregiver.

This chapter concludes with a journal entry that documents the appearance of a new symptom in Edward's early encounter with Alzheimer's disease.

Journal entry: 7/6/2019 Edward asks me to administer his eyedrops. He enters the bathroom and says, "they are on the left of the medicine cabinet, right?" I say yes, but when I see what he brings out it is a small bottle of my perfume. We laugh about it. It seems second nature; one wouldn't mistake a bottle of antifreeze for a bottle of ginger ale. The larger and more sophisticated cerebral cortex is what makes us human, differentiates us from other primates. To lose the capacity to discriminate between objects is to lose a human trait. Yet the divine spark within us is beyond this capacity and is its instigator. It is important for me to stay aware of this fact even as Edward's power of discrimination is weakening.

***

We have examined the healthy brain, and the brain damaged by Alzheimer's disease. But we need to look deeper to ascertain whether the mind is something apart from the brain. If it is, what is the relationship between brain and mind? Is the mind aware of what is happening to the brain? Deeper still is that substance or energy called consciousness. What is consciousness? What are its attributes and where does it originate? What is the relationship of brain and mind to consciousness? Is consciousness lost when the brain deteriorates, or is it invulnerable? We examine these questions next.

Chapter Two:

Brain, Mind, and Consciousness

The following are two contrasting journal entries, both from 2020, the third year of our living with Alzheimer's disease. The entries record conversations between Edward and me around the time of the presidential debates. The first shows short-term memory loss, the second also shows memory loss but adds Edward's awareness of it. Denial of the cause of his memory loss is still the barrier Edward erects to avoid full recognition of the deterioration of parts of his brain.

<u>Journal entry #1</u>: 9/30/2020: We watch the first presidential debate. We are both shocked at Trump's crudeness and rudeness. After it is over, the news anchor discusses the debate with colleagues. I ask Edward, "what did you think of the debate?".

"What debate?" he replies.

<u>Journal entry #2</u>: 11/2/2020: Edward asks me, "Who is Trump running against?" After I wait (in shock) he finally says, "Biden." He says he couldn't connect the two thoughts. I realize there was a momentary gap in his consciousness that reflected the synaptic disconnections in his brain. But I also realize that he is watching this process and willed the answer which finally came.

Later that evening, sipping wine in front of the fire, a cloud of depression descends on him. "I feel useless, empty, isolated. I can't connect even to this house – like I don't know where I am."

I press him. "You mean even the furniture, the fireplace?"

"No," he says. "I <u>feel</u> the connection, but I don't <u>know</u> the connection."

I mention Alzheimer's but he dismisses it, as he usually does, saying, "I don't feel any different than I did ten years ago."

***

A critical practice in Vedic and Buddhist teachings is to watch the mind, to watch its movements. In this way, we have some control over whether we succumb to what the Buddhists call *monkey mind* or return to the witnessing. Monkey mind is that chaotic state of mind we all experience when thoughts invade our consciousness, distracting us from the present moment. Witnessing is the practice of seeing those thoughts and then guiding the mind back to where our focus needs to be. In the above journal entry #2, Edward is watching, or witnessing, the dysfunction in his brain's ability to connect thoughts. He feels the connection but cannot verbalize it as something known. When we have difficulty associating a face with a name we are experiencing something similar to Edward's plight.

In this chapter we ask questions that are crucial to understanding the role of caregiver. These questions are:

- What is mind?
- What is mind's relationship to the brain? Are they interchangeable?
- What is consciousness?

A fundamental expression of consciousness is awareness.

Beneath awareness is the awareness of being aware. Like peeling an onion to its core, we descend into mystery.

As caregiver, I needed to find out if neuroscience and spirituality could merge and deliver truths I could accept and live by. If the brain is the origin of mind and consciousness, as some scientists believe, then the demise of the brain is a very depressing realization for the caregiver as well as the person living with Alzheimer's disease. But if consciousness is unaffected by the condition of the body and continues as soul or spiritual essence beyond death of that body, then all my efforts to assist in the care of my husband are enlightened and invigorated. I can believe those efforts will bear spiritual fruit. As Jesus says, "Let your light so shine among men that they may see your good works and glorify your Father who is in heaven."[19]

Brain and Mind

The human brain is a very sophisticated organ of the body. It houses approximately eighty-six to one hundred billion neurons (nerve cells) and one hundred trillion synapses. It is the CEO of thirty trillion cells in the body. Each cell is invested with intelligence. Studies in neuroimmunology show cells of the immune system have, like the brain, the capacity to learn and remember.[20] Even the remarkable process by which a cut on one's finger heals reveals intelligence. The brain weighs about 3 lbs. As we age the brain's volume shrinks, but whatever is learned and applied in one's life is stored and can compensate for this natural shrinkage.

The brain oversees and directs the body. The vertebrate mammalian brain developed from its early manifestation in simple invertebrates like *Aplysia*, the sea snail. The nervous system of *Aplysia* is distributed all along its ten-inch-long body to a central position in the head. In primates, and finally *homo sapiens*, the brain reaches a refined level of enlargement and complexity, especially in the frontal cortex. In the previous chapter we took a close look at the topology of the brain. Together with the brainstem and spinal cord, the parts of the brain have discrete functions that neuroscientists have defined. These parts communicate with each other through neural networks. By means of these networks, messages can be shared and activated via dendrites, axons, and neurotransmitters at synapses. This holistic schematic of communal work doesn't stop even when we sleep.

Like a corporate meeting, consensus is needed amongst the parts of the brain to act effectively. Neuroscientists have discovered that the brain can compensate when there is damage to its parts; it can adapt and be redundant. Because of the complexity of the brain, we still don't know its full capacities, nor how and by what means it develops. In the nine-month gestation of the embryo, at least 300,000 neurons are produced per minute. The brain then matures in further stages until about the age of twenty-five. During adolescence, the normal maturation of the brain is a turbulent process influenced by heredity, environment, and sex hormones. These hormones play a role in the protective myelin coating of nerve cells. Perhaps this is the reason why teenagers must wait until the sobering age of eighteen to get a driver's license. What initiates and sustains the elaborate and efficient design of the brain? Is it solely the working of natural selection based on adaptation to changing factors in the environment?

Higher brain functioning, and the behavior it elicits, refers to evolved human capacities of perception, language, memory, learning, reason, emotion, and consciousness. These capacities are modes of cognition, of mind. The thinking process can be mapped out in areas of the brain, but thoughts are subjective phenomena that we cannot see or place in the brain. Where are they? For that matter, where is mind? And what is mind? The English language has many colloquial references to the word *mind* as in *open* or *closed mind, mind over matter, mindset, changing one's mind, monkey mind* and its remedy, *mindfulness*. We say: "*I see him, in my mind's eye.*" We also say, jokingly: "*he has lost his mind.*" Where did it go? These colloquialisms suggest that we are referring to something subtle and amorphous.

Different disciplines, such as biology, psychology, and philosophy define *mind* in various ways. Definition is hard to come by with the word *mind*. The pre-Socratic Greek philosophers were much entranced with mind as the central creative force in the universe. Heraclitus (6th-5th c. BCE) described a divine Logos or Supreme Thought which disperses itself through all life forms. Anaxagoras (500-428 BCE) proposed a Universal Mind. He said that Mind is "the finest of all Things and the purest, [with] complete understanding of everything, and has the greatest power. All things which have life both the greater and the less, are ruled by Mind." [21] Mind, continues Anaxagoras, is that which moves and revolves around a still point, creating the Many from the One. Plato (428-348 BCE) called the Logos or Mind *the Good*. Eternal Ideas of material forms are contained within the Good. They receive manifest form when they enter the world of matter. The Idea of *tree*, for example, becomes a physical tree.

Plotinus (204-270 CE), the mystical Neoplatonist philosopher of Egyptian descent, added to this Platonic design the idea of a Cosmic Mind or *Nous*. The Cosmic Mind emanates from the One (or the Good) and pervades the body of the One which is the universe. The concept of the *One* is interchangeable with that of *God*.

To the scholastics of the High Middle Ages, such as Duns Scotus, this unity of life appeared as the *unus mundus*, or *one world*. In the nineteenth century, American philosopher Ralph Waldo Emerson hearkened back to the Greeks, writing in his essay, *History*, that there is a universal mind in which all humans partake. The idea of a single Whole, from which all diversified individual organisms emerge and share existence, and into which they ultimately merge, is expressed in the Hindu scripture, the *Bhagavad Gita*. Here, Krishna informs Arjuna that "He who sees the diverse forms of life, all rooted in the One, and growing forth from Him, he shall indeed find the Absolute." [22]

Renowned physicist Edwin Schrodinger believed that modern science could learn a great deal from the Greek philosophers' theories of primeval unity and cosmic mind. Physicist David Bohm appears to be borrowing from the Greeks when he proposes that the universe is constructed as a sacred web of related energies. These energies perpetually unfold into physical manifestation from an unmanifest or invisible state of being which Bohm calls the *implicate order*. This unfolding into matter, which Bohm calls the *explicate order*, is followed by an enfolding back into the unmanifest state. An image that reflects this cyclical rhythm is the ocean as it curls onto the shore and then folds into itself, retreating into the dark depths before once again rushing to shore.

The Materialist Worldview: mind as the activity of the brain

A far cry from the Greek perspective is the consensus among neuroscientists and cognitive scientists that mind emerges from the brain. This computational theory of mind asserts that mind is a product of neural processing of information by the brain. In his book *How the Mind Works,* cognitive scientist Stephen Pinker embraces this theory, arguing that thinking, and the thoughts produced, are generated by a mechanical process in the brain. This process can be studied. The Cartesian influence is evident. The French philosopher, René Descartes (1596-1650), saw the body as a machine, even as the *I* of 'I think, therefore I am' is not clearly explained. Pinker states that intelligence is the result of information patterns and the processing of correlations between pieces of information, using symbols. However, he admits that finding the source of consciousness, or awareness, in the brain is more elusive. Pinker argues that two aspects of consciousness – self-knowledge and access to information through the faculty of attention – can be explained by the computational theory of mind. But basic awareness, which Pinker calls sentience or the ability to be aware of feelings, sensations, and thoughts, is not yet understood by either computational theory or neuroscience. While mind, as a neural computer, arose as an adaptive tool to help *homo sapiens* survive through natural selection, Pinker admits that the origin of the arts, philosophy, morality, and religion is unclear. He acknowledges that existential questions like 'who am I?' and 'what happens when I die?' are difficult to reduce to biological adaptation. The source of the soaring creativity of music and art to transport the mind into a state of rapture, or the origin of the spiritual quest that makes us metaphorically reach for the stars, are unknown. If man is both a machine and a free, sentient agent, offers Pinker, then the human brain must evolve to a more advanced stage to grasp how these nonadaptive but valued aspects of human life – not to mention consciousness itself – emerge from the brain. To avoid abandoning a scientific orientation, this is the rationale available to Pinker and to most neuroscientists.

The computational theory of mind, which defines brain as the source, reflects a materialist perspective which collapses subtle mind into the physical brain. The formulation is illogical, simplistic and reductionist. For example, learning – an attribute of mind – is a lifelong, complicated, subtle process that engages cognitive faculties in various regions of the brain, as well as exterior environmental factors. Herein lies the proverbial nature/nurture confluence. How can the physical (the brain) create the subtle (the mind)? Isn't it the other way around? Because we are embodied, the subtle energy of mind works through its physical partner, the brain. The brain is the instrument by which the human mind translates into life experience creative impulses, philosophical reflections, scientific insights, musical masterpieces, mystical experiences, and inventions of tantalizing originality. Furthermore, to attribute consciousness to the creative power of the brain also defies logic. How can consciousness, which is a subtle, spiritual energy, be a child of the brain? Indian poet, Rabindranath Tagore (1861-1941), differentiates the physical from the subtle when he says: "What you are you do not see, what you see is your shadow." [23] Similarly, St. Paul encourages his followers to realize that "what is seen is temporary, but what is unseen is eternal." [24]

When we first wake up in the morning, before the awareness of 'self' and the day's lists begin, there is a brief time when there is just awareness. This awareness is not 'my' awareness. Rather, it appears as an infinite space of awareness where there is no subject, no 'me,' and therefore no desire or purpose. Quickly the ego claims this space as 'mine' and uses the energy of the universe to start the day, for 'me.' The practice of mindfulness is the effort to live every moment in the infinite space of awareness. Periods of mindful meditation teach the brain to slow down and connect with this space. The change of speed to a more restful state is reflected in brain waves. The person living with Alzheimer's disease is still in this realm of conscious energy, though he or she may have lost the ability to connect with it. It is in the infinite space of awareness that he and the caregiver, family, and friends can meet.

We must go deeper in our inquiry to find the source of mind and ultimately the source of consciousness or awareness itself. Paradoxically, we must use the reasoning power of the mind to look for the source of the mind which uses the brain to know itself. Hindu Vedanta calls this process of inquiry *vichara*. Yet even reason is not able to fully understand the origin of mind. Tagore contemplates this problem when he says: "A mind all logic is like a knife all blade. It makes the hand bleed that uses it." [25] A heightened level of consciousness or awareness is needed to discover the origin of mind. This is the level of the transcendent experiences of saints and mystics throughout the ages.

In the *Kena Upanishad,* the enquirer asks: "*'What has called my mind to the hunt? What has made my life begin? What wags in my tongue? What God has opened eye and ear?' The teacher answered: 'It lives in all that lives, hearing through the ear, thinking through the mind, speaking through the tongue, seeing through the eye.... Eye, tongue, cannot approach it nor mind know; not knowing, we cannot satisfy enquiry. It lies beyond the known, beyond the unknown. We know through those who have preached it.... That which makes the mind think but needs no mind to think, that alone is Spirit... Spirit is known through revelation.'"* [26]

Neuroplasticity

Although the perspective of neuroscience is based on the computational theory that brain creates mind, the simplistic nature of this theory is being rethought due to cutting edge research which has uncovered neuroplasticity as an attribute of the brain. Neuroplasticity is the ability of the brain to rewire itself, change its structure. As the brain develops, neurons compete for synaptic sites. Many neurons die in the process while adjacent glial cells prune and rearrange the neurons that survive at synapses to promote efficiency. Studies show that areas involved in higher brain functioning, such as memory retention and learning, can be plastic throughout life. The brain is pliable, responsive to need. For example, brain imaging studies have shown that people who are blind have auditory cells not only in the auditory area of the temporal lobe but also in the occipital lobe where the visual system operates. In nonvisual tasks such as sensory discernment of tactile or auditory stimuli, the visual cortex is active, helping its neighbor in the temporal lobe.

The question which emerges is, what directs such restructuring in the brain? In his book *Hardwiring Happiness: The New Brain Science of Contentment, Calm and Confidence,* neuropsychologist Rick Hanson uses the evidence of neuroplasticity to argue that experiences can grow the brain, rewiring its structure. Wherever the mind rests its attention, neural connections in relevant parts of the brain are thickened and increased. The positive and negative energies we create through our experiences imprint in the brain. Human evolutionary history created a negativity bias in the brain whereby painful experiences connected to survival are remembered longer than happy experiences. It is important therefore, says Hanson, to counter this hereditary bias by feeding the brain positive, calming experiences. He calls this activity *taking in the good*. Affirmations, positive visualizations, the nourishing of healthy relationships, exercise that keeps the body resilient, mindful breathing, and meditative activities reduce stress. These experiences build healthy memories as they are repeated and internalized. They return us to the natural resting state of the parasympathetic nervous system. Hanson calls this *responsive* mode of the brain *the green zone*. Its opposite, the *reactive* mode or *red zone*, is built upon the negativity bias in the brain.[27] Although this bias helped our ancestors avoid danger it is nonadaptive in a modern culture beset by chronic stress and fear. The reactive mode, stimulated through the sympathetic nervous system, should normally come in spurts, yielding to the parasympathetic nervous system's baseline of equilibrium when a threat is resolved. To minimize stress for the person living with Alzheimer's disease, the caregiver can encourage activities that take in the good to strengthen the resting state, the *green zone*.

In *Buddha's Brain: the practical neuroscience of happiness, love and wisdom*, written by Hanson in collaboration with neurologist Richard Mendius, the authors attempt to explain further the relationship of mind and brain as being in a feedback loop: change your mind, change your brain. Whatever information is fed to the brain then shapes the mind in a revolving wheel. But who or what feeds information to the brain to make the mind? The authors enter a tautological detour when they suggest that in the broadest sense mind is created by brain, body, the natural world, the cultural environment and, also, by the mind.[28] How can the mind make the mind? They acknowledge that there may be a transcendent aspect of mind that, while unprovable by science, is illuminated in great spiritual teachers, such as the Buddha. The authors acknowledge that conscious experience is not fully understood by brain science. They admit the possibility of a higher state of consciousness that is not subject to change when they advise cultivating awareness because, they affirm, it cannot be disturbed.[29]

Daniel Siegel's Deep Dive into Mind

In his book *Mind: a journey to the heart of being human*, clinical psychiatrist Daniel Siegel extends the boundaries of the concept of mind in a compelling way. Mind expands in meaning like a pebble thrown into a pond, creating concentric circles. Siegel begins with the concept in neuroscience that mind emerges from energy and information flow in the brain. There is, he asserts, a simultaneous energy exchange between mind and brain, with an instant feedback loop consistent with the fact of a mind-body continuum. The mind is embodied. He then moves to the mind's ability to self-organize in the brain. Constant self-organization is how mind enhances the brain's complexity. Mind can regulate and enhance the flow of information because self-organization is recursive; mind turns back to check on itself. The mind 'has a mind of its own.' Neuroplasticity allows the mind to change the brain's wiring, just as a computer program can be reprogrammed by the operator of the computer.

Mind is within us, says Siegel, as our *mindscape*.[30] Within us, the mind continually self-organizes towards integration, wholeness, and harmony. Siegel's assertion of mind's pursuit of wholeness is reminiscent of the conclusion Oliver Sacks arrived at in his case study of the twenty-six-year-old twins, John and Michael.[31] These young men were diagnosed as intellectually disabled, but they had an uncanny ability to 'see' numbers. Mathematics for them was not counting or calculating. They were not able to do these tasks. Their talent was a feeling for the qualities of numbers, almost a reverence for number. In one instance, when a box of matches fell to the floor and the matches scattered, the twins excitedly called out "111!" Sacks asked the twins how they counted so fast, as indeed there were 111 matches. They replied that they didn't count the matches. They 'saw' the number 111 in their minds. Sacks concluded that the twins felt the numbers vibrating within them, like tones of music, or like a contemplative vision that brought harmony to their souls. Sacks reflects on this mysterious faculty of the twins to discern numbers without counting. He proposes that this is their way to find what each of us seek: harmony and order. This search for harmony, he says, is a universal of mind.

Brain disease thwarts the flow of energy across synapses and impedes the integrative function of mind, creating either chaos or rigidity. Although Siegel doesn't mention Alzheimer's disease, both symptoms – chaos and rigidity – are endemic to Alzheimer's. In Edward's case, rigidity is seen in ever-repeating questions and in his repeated assertion that he was useless, worthless. Chaos is seen in Edward's confused state of mind caused by memory loss so that, for example, he was often unable to remember whether he ate his lunch.

Unlike some scientists, Siegel insists that subjective reality, as part of the mindscape, is real. Subjective reality develops from childhood and is stored as memories in the brain. Yes, it is not an objective fact, he admits, but it is a legitimate inclusion in any definition of mind. It follows that respecting your own and others' subjective experiences, as part of mind, is the door to interpersonal connection and harmony. *Mindsight* is Siegel's term for seeing your own mind and that of others. By recognizing and respecting another person's mindscape, healthy relationships can be forged. Siegel founded the Mindsight Institute to provide courses that help people harmonize their lives, starting with learning the science and practice of presence, or mindfulness.

The practice of staying in the present moment is fundamental to nourishing a relationship based on respect, even if the relationship is hampered on one side by Alzheimer's disease. Being present enabled me, as caregiver, to witness my own feelings and avoid the impulse to be angry or impatient. Presence reminded me of the respect due to Edward as a person as well as my husband. It isn't easy to sustain presence of mind, but when I was present I could see that his emotional life was increasingly dictated by the disease, whereas I had a choice. I was the one responsible for bringing balance and tranquility back into the relationship.

Siegel broadens his investigation of mind once again when he asserts that mind is not only private and subjective, but also relational. Mind is within us *and* between us. The 'us' includes other human beings, other life forms, and the planet itself: a *mindsphere*. We share a social mind through our culture and a planetary mind through the ecological principle of interconnectedness. Energy and information are all around us, flowing into us from cultural experiences.

What we give our attention to shapes our brains and is the impetus of neuroplasticity. As information enters our nervous systems, neurons fire. The structure of neural networks reforms in accordance with the brain's self-organizing property. Synaptic connections that hold our habits of thought and action, and glial cells, which support neurons by weaving strong myelin insulation around their axons, react to this flow of energy. Complexity is being maximized towards a refined integration.

Energy can also be produced inside the body through the power of such practices as meditation. Siegel argues that by being present and aware we can intentionally create new neural pathways. These new pathways further the goal of integration. Instead of reacting mindlessly on automatic pilot, driven by genetic and cultural habits, our minds through conscious awareness can choose how we respond. Training in mindfulness meditation specifically affects the prefrontal cortex. In turn, the PFC connects with other areas of the brain. Neural integration is thereby enhanced. Since the mind moves towards integration, individually and socially, a basic expression of this impulse is kindness and empathy. As with Hanson's counsel to *take in the good,* the social mind of healthy relationships is where science meets spirituality. Even as Alzheimer's disease challenged both Edward and me in different ways, the daily meditative practice we shared strengthened the integrative function of mind in each of us and reinforced the spiritual bond of love in our relationship.

Mind's dynamic, integrative process pushes towards wholeness. The word *whole* comes from the root *hal* meaning *healthful.* In meditation, the mind guides the brain to a state of calm; healing energy is released. Even if the brain is deteriorating due to Alzheimer's disease, healing is taking place at a subtle level, and perhaps even at a physical level.

Siegel tackles consciousness towards the end of his exploration of mind. He acknowledges that a neural correlate for consciousness (or NCC) – that is, where consciousness resides in the brain – has not yet been discovered. He agrees with certain neuroscientists who propose that the subjective experience of being aware may indicate a significant refinement in the level of integration in the brain which may, in turn, bring forth consciousness. But Siegel also acknowledges that some scientists construe consciousness as an inherent quality of the physical universe. He asks, could consciousness therefore emerge without a brain?

Using a diagram called the Wheel of Awareness, Siegel conducted an experiment to explore the possibility of the fundamental nature of consciousness. He instructed a group of people to focus their attention on the wheel in ways that moved their awareness from the rim to the hub; that is, from awareness to being aware of awareness. Participants reported a diverse set of experiences that included feelings of love, joy, peace, and the presence of God when they focused on the hub of the wheel. There was a felt sense, both bodily and psychologically, that all possibilities are at the center, the still point, which is timeless.

Resting the mind at the hub of the wheel of awareness is where the feeling of the Infinite occurs, where a direct experience of being aware of awareness is possible. Here, consciousness shows itself as a prime on the plane of infinite possibility in No-time. At the hub, says Siegel, one experiences nothing. This nothing is both full of endless potential and empty because it is *no thing*. This description of consciousness fits the Buddhist koan – *emptiness is form, form emptiness* – as well as the mystic's visionary experience of the Divine.

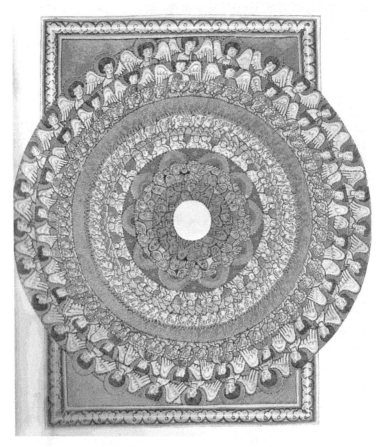

***Image 7: Mandala – Hildegard von Bingen**, 'Scivias – Wisse die Wege © Otto Müller Verlag, 9. Auflage, Salzburg 1996', used with permission*

While in a transcendent state of consciousness, 12th c. Christian mystic Hildegard de Bingen saw a mandala which she then rendered visible as art. A series of concentric circles peopled by angels and other beings surround a center hole which is empty and hollow – like a black hole, full of blinding light.

The sudden pull of the mind to this luminous center, which can happen in meditation, describes the quantum change in Edward's behavior when, for twenty minutes, he was able to transcend the disease that was rapidly destroying major parts of his brain and give an inspired class on the practice of presence. The possibility of a radical change in the capacity of the mind when it resides at this center validates the idea that consciousness is an indestructible energy, available even to a person living with Alzheimer's disease. As Krishna explains to Arjuna, "the Self, though present in all forms, retains its purity unalloyed." [32]

Consciousness: a scientific/spiritual exploration

Neuroscientists conjecture that consciousness resides in the cerebral cortex. The thalamus, as relay station of sensory experience to the cortex, aids in the production of consciousness as well as the reticular formation in the brainstem where arousal is initially felt. This may be true, but one could argue that the brain is simply reflecting, in its structure, the subtlety of mind which is, in turn, reflecting the light of consciousness which is everywhere. It is not the brain which is creating consciousness but consciousness which is creating mind and brain. As Krishna states in the *Bhagavad Gita*:

The Eternal Spirit is without beginning; neither with form nor yet without it; everywhere are its hands and feet; everywhere it has eyes that see, heads that think, mouths that speak; everywhere It listens; It dwells in all the worlds; It envelops them all. Beyond the senses, It yet shines in every sense perception. Bound to nothing, It yet sustains everything....[33]

The meaning of the word *consciousness* varies relative to the disciplines that study it, such as biology, psychology, philosophy, and spirituality. In its physical aspect, consciousness is sentience, the feeling of existence, of sensation. In its ethereal, spiritual aspect, consciousness is the God of many names and no-name. One overriding feature of consciousness is awareness. Awareness is the energy of Einstein's *unified field* and David Bohm's *implicate order* which generates and sustains the material universe. Awareness closes the gap between our constructed dualisms such as me/you or mind/body, revealing the oneness of existence. Awareness is the experience of wholeness into which all concepts of personal identity collapse. When Edward conducted the brief but potent class in philosophy, it was absent of concepts. The words flowed out of the energy of awareness. Awareness is an attribute of Spirit, or God. Krishna voices a paradox when he says in the *Bhagavad Gita*: "It [Spirit] is within all beings, yet outside; motionless yet moving; too subtle to be perceived; far away yet always near." [34]

Consciousness is not only elusive in meaning; it also appears in different forms. According to philosopher William James (1842-1910), who helped develop the discipline of psychology, rational consciousness is only one type of consciousness. In his book, *Varieties of Religious Experience*, James explores other forms of consciousness which include non-ordinary or transcendent states of consciousness. Abraham Maslow (1908-1970), pioneer in developmental psychology, builds on James' work. He argues that when basic needs are met, an individual can, by motivation and effort, reach self-actualization and even transcendence. This is the goal of meditation and contemplative prayer. As human beings, we can be aware; we can also be aware that we are aware. In those moments of self-awareness, we may realize that the self we refer to is greater than the ego, even though we cannot explain how we know this.

Hindu sage Sri Aurobindo taught his disciples that the next step in human spiritual evolution is the rediscovery of self-awareness. He calls this awareness *Supermind*. Human beings have the unique capacity of transmuting self-awareness into self-realization. As the human being becomes more conscious, the whole of Nature advances towards a realization of its hidden divinity. St. Paul suggests something similar when he says that "the whole creation groaneth and travaileth in pain," together with humans, for new birth in Christ. [35] The metaphor is that of childbirth.

Let's do an experiment. Become aware of your body and your physical surroundings. Take it all in through the mind's faculty of attention. Give time to observe it all: sounds, sights, smells, and sensations of the body like breathing. Recognize that the movements in mind – the thoughts that fire in the brain – are, for the moment, quiescent because our attention is occupied with being aware through the senses. We are sensorily aware. With our eyes open, we see material forms in space. These forms appear separate from each other. From childhood, the brain is imprinted with the idea that the material forms we see are separate and different from each other. An illusory worldview – called *maya* in Hindu Vedanta – is built on this impression. Now, close the eyes.... Did awareness leave when we closed our eyes? No, awareness remains. There's just no content, and no separate forms. Even if thoughts enter and exit the mind, they do so within this unchanging ground of awareness. We are witnessing awareness and being awareness at the same time. With eyes closed, we may be more aware of our breathing because with sight gone the other senses, such as touch, are heightened. Sufism teaches that the source of Creation is the breath of God. The universe, God's body, breathes. The Hebrew word for *soul* is *nephesh* which also means *breath*. When we breathe it is God that breathes through us. Our souls rest in that breath.

Connection with this unitary consciousness is both a knowing and a sensation. Our minds cognize this awareness; our bodies feel it, as if through the pores of the skin. Even the neurons in our brains are talking to each other, at synapses, reflecting an elemental interconnectedness of all life forms. Everything is arising from consciousness and falling back into consciousness in a continuous oscillation of manifestation and dissolution. We are born into consciousness, sustained by consciousness, and return to consciousness.

The primary role of consciousness aligns with the indestructible nature of spirit, of soul, which is unaffected by the brain's deterioration. If both the person who lives with Alzheimer's disease and the caregiver can tap into this unifying consciousness they will feel their connection to each other. This sensation of unity will repel the rise of negative emotions which can occur in difficult situations.

As the disease progresses, and the neural circuits at synapses are increasingly severed by toxic proteins, the person living with Alzheimer's will feel more and more isolated. This feeling of isolation creates anxiety. In response, the caregiver will need to rely on providing more physical contact through touch and more comfort through loving words.

In the second journal entry at the top of this chapter, Edward states that he "*felt* the connection but didn't *know* the connection" between two pieces of information. Similarly, even without a damaged brain, we may sometimes feel a connection to the All, but we don't fully know it because the content of the mind is full of filters that prevent illumination.

Emerson speaks of immersion in Nature as a powerful means of dispersing these filters and revealing pure consciousness as our true nature. He writes in the essay *Nature*:

Standing on the bare ground – my head bathed by the blithe air and uplifted into infinite space – all mean egotism vanishes. I become a transparent eyeball. I am nothing. I see all; the currents of the Universal Being circulate through me; I am part or parcel of God.[36]

To *feel* 'the currents of the Universal Being' circulating through us is both a physical sensation and an indication of emotional intelligence. The prefrontal cortex and amygdala in the brain are key players in this type of intelligence. In Daniel Goleman's seminal book *Emotional Intelligence,* he argues that human beings possess two interconnected intelligences: rational and emotional. They spring from the same biological root. The neocortex develops out of a more primitive emotional storehouse of experience lodged in the limbic system. The limbic system grows out of the olfactory lobe which investigates the world by means of the oldest sense – smell. This original role of the senses suggests the preeminence of sensory awareness as the route towards feeling universal consciousness. In caring for the person living with Alzheimer's disease, emphasis can be given to finding ways that accentuate his or her sensory connection to the natural environment. For example, walking together in a park, with the attention out, it is possible to feel exhilarated and soothed by sights and smells of the natural world. Instead of feeling isolated, the person with Alzheimer's disease feels connected both to his companion and to the world around him.

The phenomenon of light is an apt metaphor for consciousness. Though invisible and subtle, light is physically everywhere, sustaining life through the energy rays of the sun. In the Kabbalah of Jewish mysticism, it is written that *Ein Sof*, the Unnameable, sent down from heaven emanations of light. These emanations were transformed into matter and became the Creation. Mind, in its dual capacities of rational and emotional intelligence, can be enlightened by the light of consciousness when brought to quietude, as in deep meditation. At such times, mind knows itself as the light. In the Allegory of the Cave, in Plato's *Republic*, prisoners sit chained in the darkness of a cave watching shadows of people and objects pass along a wall in front of them. The shadows are lit by a fire behind the prisoners who believe these shadows to be reality. When one of the men is released and guided out of the cave he is blinded by the light of the sun. He has difficulty accepting the new illuminated world to be real, so steeped is he in delusory beliefs.

The erroneous beliefs we hold about ourselves and the world veil this inner light within us. When cognitive scientist Stephen Pinker is stymied by the puzzle of how consciousness emerges from the brain, he advances the idea that human beings at this evolutionary stage are not yet equipped to understand this process. Yet mystics over the ages have understood. They experienced visions of Divine Light as the true reality because they lifted their minds to higher states of consciousness. Julian of Norwich, fifteenth century English anchoress, describes her visions as *showings* – revelations of God's love. Such subjective experiences are no less credible than empirical findings, if one accepts subjective experience as a legitimate part of the mind, as Daniel Siegel does.

The *Bhagavad Gita* uses the metaphor of light to describe the Eternal Spirit who is "the Light of lights, beyond the reach of darkness... the Presence in the hearts of all." [37] If we consider the mind in both its rational and emotional aspects, then the heart is also a discerner of truth. The heart is the site of compassion and love. It feels the connections to all life. Anthropologist Edward Tylor reported that while doing field work with an indigenous tribe he asked a tribal member where he thought the mind was located. The man put his hand over his heart. We make this gesture when we refer to ourselves.

The intelligence of the heart is receptive and yielding. Paradoxically, because the heart offers no resistance, it is protected by its very vulnerability. The heart disperses love indiscriminately and transmutes into love whatever negative energy it may receive. The heart intuits what is real at the subtle level. The *Katha Upanishad* says, "God, the inmost Self, no bigger than a thumb, lives in the heart."

³⁸ An important practice for the caregiver is to keep her own heart open and yielding, especially when the person living with Alzheimer's disease cannot control his own heart's reactions, which often devolve into anger and resentment.

In *Dark Night of the Soul,* sixteenth century Christian mystic, St. John of the Cross, describes a light that burned in his heart. The light guided him through the secret and solitary darkness of contemplation where he prayed that God would purge the imperfections in his soul, revealing its intrinsic light. If Alzheimer's disease is a creeping darkness in which the light of the mind and brain is gradually obscured, this does not mean that there is no light in the body. Nor is the light absent from the mind and heart. It is merely hidden. The task of the caregiver and family is to remember and uncover that light within the stricken loved one. Thirteenth century Sufi poet, Jalaluddin Rumi, tells us what to do. He writes: "Don't turn your head. Keep looking at the bandaged place. That's where the light enters you." [39]

The story of Jacques Lusseyran, related in his memoir *And There Was Light,* elucidates Rumi's counsel. It is the inner light of consciousness which Lusseyran experiences when, at eight years old, he becomes blind from an accident at school. Lusseyran writes that he learned to rely on sound and touch to orient him to his surroundings, but, more importantly, he found that he could 'see' objects and people around him by feeling their pressure as they came closer to him.[40] He could thus navigate the geography around him. Moreover, he found that his sense of interconnectedness to and respect for every living being was heightened by this inner light. He learned that communion with his environment was lessened when he was afraid or tried to grasp things. Then the isolation of the blind closed him in. He describes the loss of sight as abundantly compensated for by the gift of inner vision. This gift may, he says, be related to an opening of the third eye. According to esoteric literature, the third eye of insight and intuition is located between the eyebrows.

Lusseyran learned braille shortly after he became blind. He was an exemplary student. At the age of seventeen, while engaged in study at the elite schools of France, Germany invaded and occupied his country. The year was 1939. World War II was underway. He became involved in the French Resistance movement as the leader of 600 boys. These youths entrusted Lusseyran with the task of recruiting members because of his uncanny ability to 'read' people as to their loyalty or treachery. Towards the end of the war, he was captured and sent to Buchenwald concentration camp where he spent over a year in filthy, inhumane conditions. He was able to avoid depression and madness, which afflicted many of his comrades in the camp, by focusing his mind on hearing and distributing accurate news of the war and by offering hope and healing to those in need. He acknowledges that, had he not kept his attention on the needs of others, instead of on his own ego, he may not have survived. Lusseyran was one of the few prisoners who survived Buchenwald.

The relevance of Lusseyran's life to our examination of Alzheimer's disease is this: even with a severe physical impairment the inner light of consciousness is still functional. It is impervious to physical limitations.

Consciousness and modern physics

Two discoveries in modern physics – the wave-particle complementarity principle and non-locality – reveal the primacy of consciousness. In 1905, in his Special Theory of Relativity, Einstein broke through the mechanical laws of classical physics. Through the mathematical equation $E=mc2$ (energy equals mass times the speed of light squared) he showed that matter and energy are essentially the same. They just appear in two different forms. Following Einstein's work, physicists began to discover new laws, at atomic and subatomic levels, that govern the shaping of energy and matter. When Max Planck discovered that heat radiation delivers its energy in packets, and not in a continuous stream, he was recognizing a bizarre property of light and matter to appear as both energy particle and wave. He named these fundamental but strangely amoebic energy capsules *quanta*. When Niels Bohr researched the superficially discrete boundaries of matter, he saw these boundaries dissolve at atomic and subatomic levels, revealing the fundamental indivisibility of energy. An intricate, non-linear energy matrix of particle-waves sketched dance-like patterns of energy exchange and relationship. Common distinctions, like animate versus inanimate matter, became fuzzy. Bohr's discovery of the wave and particle appearances of the electron as complementary properties became known as the complementarity principle.

Werner Heisenberg added another mind-blowing discovery. He found that electrons display themselves as waves or particles, not in a dualistic way, but depending upon their environment. The scientist who is conducting an experiment is not a subject working on an object. Rather, he is a part of the environment, of the whole. Therefore, his presence influences whether the electron appears as a wave or a particle. When a quantum object is measured by the scientist, it appears in a local spot as a particle. When left alone the object spreads like a wave, existing simultaneously in various places. The fact that the observer, in this case the scientist, is not separate from what is observed – as in a subject-object dichotomy – establishes a radically new worldview. Interconnectedness and interdependence are revealed. Life forms are not objects in a mechanistic universe. Life forms, including our own, are part of a great animate web of life, an organic whole from the smallest atom to the galaxies. That whole is consciousness, which in turn creates both the material world and the world of mental phenomena. This information is important for the caregiver to absorb. To realize her subtle connection to the person she is caring for will infuse her words and actions with empathy and patience. She will know in experience the words of Krishna when he says to Arjuna that Spirit "is in all beings undivided, yet living in division."[41]

The holographic model of the universe backs up the evidence of an interconnected, conscious universe. Using a special type of lensless photography, it was found that when a holographic photo is taken (of a tree, for example) and a section of the photo (such as the trunk) is cut out and then enlarged, the enlarged photo will show not an enlarged trunk but the whole tree. The hologram reveals two principles: the whole is greater than the sum of the parts and the whole is contained in every part. The science of holography arose out of the work of philosopher-scientist Arthur Koestler. He coined the word *holon* to stand for each individual thing in nature. A holon is a whole unto itself but also part of a larger whole. Thus, each of us is an individual, but also a member of society and a part of the natural world. The natural world is, in turn, a part of the organism of the planet.

At the microcosmic level, each nerve cell is a holon within the brain which is a holon of the body. In 1969, Karl Pribram, a neurophysiologist at Stanford University, suggested that the brain may operate like a hologram, with bioelectric frequencies showing themselves throughout the brain. Thus, for example, memory may not be relegated only to a specific locale, the temporal lobe. The act of remembering and storing memories may spread in wavelike frequency patterns along nerve cell networks in the whole brain. Pribram's hypothesis supports the more recent evidence in neuroscience of neuroplasticity. The holographic model introduces a question: might the deterioration of the brain in people living with Alzheimer's disease be halted in a way that preserves the capacity of the brain to use compensatory measures to restore its functioning?

Mathematical models that chart chaotic systems show hidden patterns of order within the chaos. In the 1970s, Belgian chemist Ilya Prigogine built on this discovery with the idea of autocatalysis. Autocatalysis is the inherent inclination of living systems to move from equilibrium into instability, in order to regenerate at a more adaptive and life-enhancing level of existence. When disease strikes the body, the impulse towards this regenerative phase is activated. In this way the body may recover and return to health. If not, and death ensues, the regenerative impulse becomes the means towards transformation into a new structure. In spiritual terms, the soul departs to continue its evolution in a new body. Based on Prigogine's research, might the chaotic energy in the Alzheimer brain be transmuted into a regenerative, life-enhancing phase, perhaps through drugs not yet invented? This regenerative work would complement the mind-brain's own self-organizing capacity towards ever-refined integration. The capacity for self-organization is known as *autopoiesis*. Each individual organism maximizes its structural integrity by maintaining and enhancing its structure in the will to live.

Non-locality is another evidence of the seamless, all-inclusive nature of consciousness. All life forms are interconnected and thus can communicate with each other. They are, together, the cosmic subject, the non-local consciousness itself. We have mistakenly identified with a version of the cosmic subject that we create – our own small ego and its mind-brain which is separate from other mind-brains. An experiment with elementary particles, conducted by French physicist Alain Aspect in 1982, reveals the truth of non-local consciousness. In the experiment, two identical photons were released by a calcium atom. Although they went in opposite directions, there was communication between them. If one photon was tweaked in a certain way, the other photon, though at some distance, was affected and behaved in synchrony.

Quantum non-locality is also found in ordinary experiences, as when we think of someone and immediately receive a call from that person. Telepathy, or distant viewing, is communication by means of non-local consciousness. Because the brain is a physical organ limited and localized in space-time, how can the brain generate instances of non-local consciousness? The function of the mind-brain is clear: through its connection to the senses, it can study and understand reality in its material aspect *within* non-local consciousness.

Although studies have proven the validity of telepathy, in both psychic and non-psychic subjects, the materialist perspective looks askance at such studies. They appear to throw the orderly world of causality into incomprehensible chaos. This conclusion is inaccurate. Non-local consciousness occurs at a higher dimension, or frequency, than Newton's mechanical laws of cause and effect. Those laws still hold at the level where they operate. According to an experiment conducted by Mexican neurophysiologist Jacobo Grinberg-Zylberbaum and his colleagues, human mind-brains communicate just as photons do at a distance. In the experiment, two subjects interact for about thirty minutes until they begin to feel a direct connection with each other. They then enter separate enclosures that block all electromagnetic signals. The brain of one of the subjects is stimulated by a light signal. As the subjects continue to mentally nurture a sensitivity to each other, the light appears to transfer itself into the unstimulated brain which shows telltale electrophysiological activity.

The Institute of Noetic Sciences, founded in 1973 by astronaut and visionary Edgar Mitchell, is dedicated to research that explores non-local properties of consciousness. On the return trip of Apollo 14 to Earth in 1971, Mitchell had a transpersonal experience that changed his life. As he gazed out the window of the spacecraft at the stars and the home planet where he was headed, Mitchell experienced a transcendent lift of mind and spirit. He felt the interconnectedness of all bodies and realized that the universe was conscious, intelligent, harmonious, and full of love. This epiphany redirected his life's mission.

The work of the Institute examines evidence of

transcendent and/or altered states of consciousness. This evidence contradicts the materialist worldview that the brain, a physical substrate of complex neurons, generates consciousness. Rather, combining science, particularly quantum physics, with spirituality, the Institute proposes a more holistic model of consciousness that validates subjective, phenomenological experiences of noesis. Noesis refers to cognition through the direct experience of reality. Meditation, for example, can yield intuitive knowledge that all phenomena, interior and exterior, are in consciousness and thus interconnected. Just because the experience cannot be empirically validated does not mean it is fraudulent. As Hamlet told Horatio: "There are more things in heaven and Earth, Horatio, / than are dreamt of in your philosophy." [42]

In a 2022 article written by the director of the Institute of Noetic Sciences and her colleagues, this new paradigm of scientific thought is outlined.[43] Of relevance to this book's objective, which is to understand whether consciousness continues as a backdrop in Alzheimer's disease, the authors cite well-documented cases of people whose cognitive awareness remains, even as the brain is severely damaged by disease. Terminal lucidity is a phenomenon that suggests that, though awareness is embodied, it may not be solely dependent on the brain due to the non-physical, non-local properties of consciousness. The fact that Edward could conduct a class in an astute manner, even as his diseased brain was rapidly deteriorating, was a sign of a hidden, healthy dimension of consciousness. Patients with a terminal neurodegenerative disease – such as Alzheimer's – have been reported to display normal cognitive functions, even mental clarity, shortly before death. In one case a patient, whose cancer had metastasized to the brain, destroying most of the brain tissue, regained awareness an hour before his death and held a conversation with family members for about five minutes before passing. The authors report that though terminal lucidity defies what we know from neuroscience and neuroanatomy, instances of it have been reported for over 250 years.[44]

The work of the Institute of Noetic Sciences is aimed at a paradigm shift that redirects the scientific trajectory away from 'brain creates mind and consciousness' to its flip side, 'consciousness creates mind creates brain.' In this inversion we revisit the worldview of Greek philosophy, the mystical experiences at the heart of all religions, and the ancient scriptures from the East.

In the *Bhagavad Gita*, the god-man Krishna defines the light of consciousness as the Self. This Self creates and sustains matter. Krishna says:

The body of man is the playground of the Self. That which knows the activities of Matter sages call the Self. I am the Omniscient Self that dwells in the playground of Matter.[45]

Tutored by this new paradigm, we can acknowledge the underside of events of which we are usually only dimly aware. We can become more sensitive to the non-physical, non-local properties of consciousness. This sensitivity flowers when the mind is connected to the senses, and we live inside the moment. At such fertile times, our minds are open to a confluence of events. This phenomenon is called synchronicity. Like Alice who falls into the rabbit hole, locates the key, and enters wonderland, we may, through synchronicity, experience a quantum nonlocal collapse of space/time. The following example of such an experience occurred when I was writing this chapter. It taught me the truth of non-local consciousness.

In August 2023, four months after Edward's death, I went to Saratoga Springs for a few days. Edward and I used to go there around the time of our wedding anniversary, August 19th. We would stay in a bed and breakfast inn near the center of town, enjoy the Roosevelt baths, take in a concert at SPAC, and, early in the morning, watch the horses work out at the Saratoga Racetrack. I wanted to revisit the places where we spent time, starting with a picnic lunch at Saratoga Springs Park. I sat on the same bench where we sat and began to eat my lunch. The brick buildings housing the historic Roosevelt baths were diagonally across from me. It was a sunny day, and as I ate, I watched people walk their dogs and listened to the sound of lawn mowers as park employees mowed the vast stretches of green grass. Suddenly I felt a sharp pain in my left ankle. Three years ago, I broke the ankle on the third day of our visit to Saratoga Springs, but since then the ankle had fully healed. The accident occurred near the geysers which were down the hill from the baths, not far from where I was now sitting, maybe one-quarter mile away. I tried to relax and will the pain away, but it only increased. I wondered how I was going to walk back to the car. I didn't want to reinjure the ankle. I quickly finished eating, carefully rose from the bench, and slowly limped back to where the car was parked, trying to put as little weight on the left foot as possible. Once in the car, I gently massaged the ankle and waited. Finally, as I left the park and drove towards the main part of town, the symptoms of the injury began to lessen. I was able to walk a few blocks on Broadway; my ankle held up. I then drove to the bed and breakfast and checked in.

Once in my room, I sat and reflected on what had happened in the park. There was no residue of pain. It was as if the incident hadn't happened. The sensation of pain seemed to come out of nowhere. It was as if the body, and specifically the ankle, was aware of where I was geographically and 'remembered' the injury. The past entered the present in conjunction with the space of the place where the ankle had been injured three years ago. There was a space-time collapse in which a singular truth was being revealed: we are all embedded in the energy of non-local consciousness. The brain was the localized site of the memory – specifically the prefrontal cortex and hippocampus, perhaps mediated by the entorhinal cortex which is the gateway for information flowing to and from the hippocampus. According to recent research, the entorhinal cortex may also participate in sensory perception. The brain and ankle were sensing the place and remembering a particularly memorable incident that triggered the negativity bias of the brain that registered pain by means of the senses. The brain and ankle were communicating through the neural circuits in the body, but their physical roles were enclosed in the larger whole of non-local consciousness.

In the next chapter we consider time in its linear aspect and what happens when, through the degenerative process of Alzheimer's disease, a person is trapped in the dominance of the present tense.

Chapter Three:

Dominance of the Present Tense

Being present, and sustaining that presence, undergirds all spiritual practice. The art of presence is also called mindfulness. The benefits of mindfulness are many. Being mindful we enjoy life more, even in simple ways, like savoring the taste of an apple picked right off the tree. When we are mindful, we are more responsive to others because our attention is on listening to what our companion is saying, instead of rehearsing what we will say in response. Rather than reacting to events, we learn to respond with detachment and reasonableness. Mindfulness helps us exercise the brain, conserve energy, buffer the constant intrusion of information in our fast-paced, digital culture, and even find inner peace at times of conflict or sorrow.

When Edward conducted work parties at The School of Practical Philosophy (hereafter referred to as The School), he taught students how to rest the attention on the work they were engaged in. This mental effort demands presence. In hammering a nail into wood, for example, the attention is directed to the space where the point of the nail is entering the wood. The mind likes to play, but it also likes to be disciplined and attentive to a task. So, the instruction to be given, when the mind becomes distracted by extraneous thoughts, is to acknowledge the diversion and bring the mind back to the work at hand – without self-recrimination. Attention is key to any work. When baking a cake, it doesn't do to forget the baking powder because your mind darted away to imagining preparations for a party. When mowing the lawn, a slip in the attention could erase a flower bed.

One of the first signs of Alzheimer's disease is short-term memory loss, due to the erosion of temporal lobe functions. Particularly affected is the hippocampus, the major site of memory. One might conclude that this loss is a gift rather than a curse as it places the mind squarely in the present moment. But the erasure of each moment as it passes through the mind is abnormal because the past is in the present. Time is a human construct. Past, present, and future is a continuum in the stream of timeless consciousness. Associations from the past saturate impressions in the present. Even as we practice attention in the moment, presence has an invisible backdrop of past moments. The five senses of smell, taste, sight, sound, and touch are instrumental in eliciting memory. Remembrance of their potency is layered in the brain by countless neural networks that are active 24/7. A robin's song in early spring can bring back childhood memories of watching birds return from their winter homes. The feel of leaves underfoot in fall can remind us of times we walked with loved ones on forest paths. If we want to retrieve a memory from the past to enrich the present moment, we can do so. The process of the past resurfacing in the present usually happens automatically – sometimes chaotically. The purpose of mindfulness is to bring the habitual circus of our mind's chatter under control.

Pythagoras (570-490 BCE) was a Greek philosopher, mathematician, and scientist. He also founded a spiritual school. Legend has it that he advised his disciples to make an inventory of each day's activities before going to sleep.

The objective of the practice was to see how much they remembered of the day. This recalling of the past in the present would show how conscious they had been. Where there was slippage in memory, the disciples would reaffirm in their journaling a commitment to improving their practice of presence.

A person living with Alzheimer's disease is deprived of the security of this inner clock of past, present, and future. The 'now' is fleeting and thin, as each moment is removed from memory. It might feel like walking on the edge of a precipice, each step being a moment that falls over the cliff; or it might feel like an acrobat who is walking a tightrope without a net underneath. Each step is precarious. Such an experience is not only disorienting, but also frightening. A generalized anxiety pervades the psyche. Edward experienced this anxiety about memory loss but, in the early stages, it wasn't coming from an acknowledgement that he had Alzheimer's disease. He was mystified and confused about not remembering simple things, like whether he put honey in his tea, but he chalked it up to age. The defense mechanism of denial went into gear once his condition was diagnosed. Denial shielded him from overt admission of his sickness and the fear that can accompany such admission.

David's wife, Karen, developed early onset Alzheimer's disease in 2014 at age sixty-three. She was a psychotherapist, proud of her cognitive faculties and the fact that she was helping many people, particularly those with dissociative identity disorder. When she became aware that she was forgetting appointments and overbooking them she became anxious, knowing that her behavior was unusual. After being diagnosed with Alzheimer's disease four years later in 2018, her professional integrity did not allow her to deny the diagnosis; she knew it to be true. Watching her short-term memory disappear, Karen went into a tailspin of fear and anger. As the disease intensified, denial attached itself to these emotions.

Reverend Diane Epstein serves as a chaplain at the Hudson Valley Hospice. She is also an interfaith minister. She told me that some of the patients she sees with advanced Alzheimer's disease go through a phase in which they display a demeanor of peaceful passivity. They have forgotten the very memory loss that afflicts them. Rather like a baby whose history is yet to be written, the person living with Alzheimer's disease lives in a fleeting present, unperturbed, at least superficially. At the same time, it is important to remember that even if the person living with Alzheimer's disease appears childlike, he or she is an adult, with a full life of experience, even if the memory of that experience remains out of reach.

In Jean-Paul Sartre's play *No Exit,* three people – two women and a man – are escorted by a valet into a Second-Empire French drawing room where they are to live. The furnishings are sparse. There are three velveteen sofas in different colors. A huge bronze sculpture sits on the mantelpiece. The door is locked. There are no windows. It gradually becomes evident to the three residents, as well as to the reader, that they are in hell. Their 'sins' are revealed during the play. The man, Garcin, is afraid that they will be tortured; but torture is what they do to each other. They are new to hell so they can still see and hear some of what is happening on earth. They are forever entombed in the stuffy, airless drawing room with only their masks to deal with – their hidden agendas, fears, and anxieties. The stigma associated with Alzheimer's disease, as with all types of dementia, is due to the fear in each of us that we may become trapped in a body without an operating, normal mind. This place of mental-emotional confinement is like Sartre's drawing room. There is no exit. It is like Dante's inferno where "those who have lost the good of intellect" lament their fate.[46]

Journal Entries

The following selected journal entries span the early years of Edward's life with Alzheimer's disease, from 2019 to 2021. They show a gradual fraying of memory. They mark Edward's entrance into *No Exit*.

2019

8/14: "Let's visit Asheville when we leave Florida to come home," I say.

Edward says, "Been there, done that."

The next minute he says, "Why don't we visit Asheville?"

10/2: A window-washing company is working here today. I ask Edward to put the screens back up when they finish, while I go out to shop. When I get home Edward says he got confused and couldn't find the screens. We look for them. Then I see that the screens are in the windows.

10/25: Edward leaves the water running in the bathroom sink twice. He washes dishes, including the brass candle holder.

2/18: Edward has a bowl of ice cream. One hour later,

he gets another helping. I say, "you already had a bowl."

"Did I?" he asks.

2020

3/6: Lunch with old friends, Irv and Pat. Edward gets excited by an exchange with Pat about meditation, but otherwise he is quiet. On the way home, he asks, "Who were they?" When I say they are old friends, that we visited them in Ocala, he remembers their house but not their faces nor facts of their lives.

4/12: Easter Sunday. Covid is raging. Edward is steady but memory is going. We meditate, then he asks, a few minutes later, "Did we meditate? Are you ready to meditate?"

6/17: I ask him to tighten a doorknob and vacuum the car. He does the first task but forgets the second. I must give him one job at a time.

7/23: Tough day for Edward. He needs to vacuum because of a flare-up in my lower back. He gets very tired, feels victimized, forgets where to plug in the cord. Before supper, he pours me red wine instead of white and pours white for himself. He says it doesn't matter to him. I say it matters to me. He becomes distant and defensive which is a cover for his knowing and fearing his memory loss.

He asks the year: "Is it 1986 or 2086?"

"Don't you know?" I ask.

"No." He smiles guiltily, "I don't know."

"It's 2020," I say.

He nods. "Right, 2020."

8/12: For supper we have corn. He tells me to butter mine first, which I do. Passing the butter to him, he says, "You need to butter yours too, don't you?"

I say, "I already did." I add the words, "don't you remember?" Big mistake. This is not a helpful response; I have to stop saying it.

After supper, he has a meltdown. He gets frustrated and ultra-sensitive. Outbursts continue as we watch the news, but when he settles down and speaks in a calm tone, I think he is ashamed. I feel ashamed too, that I made him aware of his memory loss.

9/9: We watch TV news for six hours straight. When I mention highlights of the main stories, he says, "what stories?" Information comes in and immediately deletes itself. I am still giving him piano lessons. Each lesson disappears into the black hole of forgetting. We persevere because it is a good mind-body exercise. I think he is aware that his mental faculties are fading. I must be careful to repeat my answers with kindness and stay present no matter how many times he asks the same questions. We walk out to get the mail after supper. As we head back, he asks, "did we get the mail?" I show him the mail in my hand, then hold his hand as we walk back to the house.

11/4: We are at the doctor's office for blood work. When the nurse asks Edward questions, I start to talk for him. He stops me. "I'll speak for myself," he says. I stop, but then when the nurse asks why he is there he says, "for an annual physical."

I intervene. I say, "no, it's about bloodwork." He needs

to feel independent. He is afraid of losing control.

12/14: We go to Newburgh to get an ultrasound on his kidneys and do errands. Coming home, he is quiet. I ask him if he is ok. He says he feels disoriented because of all the stops we are making. I am realizing how taxing it is for people living with Alzheimer's to absorb, organize, and remember new information. The self-organizing property of the brain is disrupted. This disruption leads to his feeling disoriented. The brain can't keep pace with the moment-to-moment influx of information. That influx is the source of a sense of continuity and security. It's what grounds us. Edward is floating in space. He's living a play whose scenes are mixed up; he can't follow the plot.

2021

1/3: Breaking news about Trump trying to intimidate the GA secretary of state. We are both shocked. In the immediate present, Edward connects clearly to the incident; the emotive component in his brain (amygdala) is triggered. But in leaving that environment, in going downstairs, he doesn't retain the content, just the feeling that something is wrong.

4/1: Before bed he asks four times, with fifteen seconds in between, "should I wear socks to bed?"

4/3: We're back from two weeks in Florida. It's Easter Saturday. We call Dolores, his sister, and they talk. As they finish their conversation he says to me, "I didn't know where I was; I felt strange."

"Where did you think you were?" I ask.

"At Mum's house."

Time away on a vacation has blurred his memory of this house. He asks me continually where things are. "It's familiar and yet unfamiliar – a lack of connection," he says.

4/28-30: Edward's brother, Ludge, died a week ago and we are driving to Pittsburgh with our sons, John and James, for the funeral. When we go to the wake, Edward doesn't recognize his niece, Christina, Ludge's daughter. He feels disoriented. When we return home he says, "we've come from a different country."

5/2: Today is a long, odd day. A sequence of conversations shows memory loss and physical disorientation that indicates damage to the proprioceptive sense of the body in space. When Edward comes downstairs in the morning, I ask him if he took his pills.

"No," he says.

"Did you shower?" I ask.

"No." It turns out he did both, but he forgot. At lunch I tell him I talked with Christina to see how she is faring. He seems confused. "Christina?" he says.

"Do you know who she is?" I ask. He pauses to think.

"She's my—" There is a blank in the conversation. I fill in.

"Niece," I say. Then I ask, as non-threatening as I can, "And who is her father?"

"I don't know," he says.

"Ludge," I say. "He died and we went to the funeral."

"I know he died," he says testily.

"Do you remember where we went for the funeral?" I ask.

"South America?" he offers.

"We went to Pittsburgh, where you grew up. Do you remember Ludge's house?"

"I don't remember where it is. Describe it for me," he says. I describe it but it doesn't register. He voices surprise that he can't remember.

"I'm not crazy yet," he says.

"You're not crazy, your memory is going, that's all," I say.

Later at supper he says something he is increasingly saying, as if he is watching what is happening to him. "I feel like I'm nowhere. I can't connect."

It is as if pieces of memories and even present experiences must constantly be reassembled and put in order, so they make sense, like a puzzle. The healthy brain does this self-organizing in nanoseconds.

5/25: Edward continues to forget his morning routine. While I am out grocery shopping he gets up earlier than usual. He leaves one of the stove burners on. This is worrisome. His movements are getting awkward. We need to find a one-story house without stairs.

9/4: I mention our older son John's birthday coming up. "John's a year older than me," Edward says.

Stunned, I say, "John is your son, how can he be older?"

He looks mystified. "You are confusing him with Ludge," I say. This has happened before. He nods and laughs.

"Why did I say that?" he muses.

9/9: We drive down to John's house for his birthday. Edward doesn't recognize the house. He asks if John and Magda (his wife) are married. When we return home, he says he feels disoriented and tired. He goes to bed early.

11/12: There is a lot of disorientation and confusion this evening along with fatigue (sundown syndrome). Edward asks questions before we get into bed:

"Are we married?" he asks, tentatively, as if he is sleeping next to me out of wedlock.

"Yes," I reply.

"Am I losing my mind? I didn't know we were married," he says, straight-faced. "How long have we been married?"

"Fifty-four years," I say, as I turn down the covers.

"My brain feels scrambled," he says. "I know John and James, but I didn't know they were our sons." A pause. "Is Ludge dead?"

I nod. "Yes."

"I didn't know," he says. "Was there a funeral?"

"Yes," I say. "We went to the funeral."

"I know there is a decline," he says; "and it gets worse."

He is referring to Alzheimer's disease, but he can't say

the word. He is still reluctant to accept the fact that he has the disease. I turn out the light and press my hand against his as we lay in bed. I wipe my cheek as the tears come.

11/25: We go to James' house for Thanksgiving. On the way home he asks, "where were we?"

"Your son James' house," I say.

"Have we been there before?" he asks.

"Many times," I reply.

"Why did we go?" he asks.

"For Thanksgiving," I say. A pause.

"Are we married? How old am I?"

2022

1/10: I light a candle at every dinner to make it special. At the table, Edward waxes philosophical about losing his memory. I feel how depressed it is making him. "There's the past, but I have no desire to recall it," he says. "The future doesn't exist – no expectations. Just the present, regulated by habit. Like eating. I have no desire to eat but I go at the food out of habit, like an animal." Nothing seems to give him joy anymore. In the dark and cold of winter it's even hard to appreciate Nature. The rays of the sun coming in the window, birds at the feeder: he doesn't notice these small delights. He is spending more time dozing in his wing-back chair.

1/28: We go out to dinner and a movie with James and his family. On the way home, Edward says, "You better hang on to the keys to give them back."

"What do you mean?" I ask.

"To the person who owns this car," he says.

"We own it," I say.

"Really? Since when?"

"Over a year," I say. He laughs.

***

As the tissue of the hippocampus, and other areas of the brain involved in memory, decay, the vacuum created by short-term memory loss begins to spread into other forms of loss. Lost is the ability to recognize people we have known for many years, even relatives. Places once familiar become unfamiliar. The journal entries above indicate these successive losses. Eventually memory loss can affect one's sense of self. Oliver Sacks describes the case of Mr. T. who had a severe case of memory loss, called Korsakov syndrome. This is a neural degeneration of the mammillary bodies which are on the underside of the hypothalamus, close to the brainstem. They are also closely connected to the hippocampus. In its simplest form, Korsakov syndrome arises from chronic alcohol misuse. Mr. T. was unable to remember anything for more than a few seconds. Continually disoriented and amnesiac, Mr. T. was in a continual frenzy, fabricating all kinds of fictitious information about himself. Because he could not remember a real-life subjective world as his identity, Mr. T had to compulsively create pseudo-narratives to maintain some sense of self. Awareness of his condition compelled him to concoct and replace story after story to compensate for having no story of his own.

Another case of Korsakov syndrome that Sacks describes is that of Jimmie, a former Navy man who served in World War II. A drinking problem accentuated his memory loss. He could remember nothing that happened to him after the year 1945. Sacks wondered if Jimmie had anything in his current life that gave him emotional meaning and comfort, anything which indicated that his soul was alive and nourished. He knew that Jimmie attended Mass regularly. When he asked the sisters at the chapel whether they thought Jimmie's soul survived the abyss of amnesia, they exclaimed, "watch him at Mass!" Sacks did so; he saw an aura of peace envelop Jimmie's whole demeanor. He saw the same peace when Jimmie was contemplating nature or listening to fine music. Sacks concluded that while empirical science can diagnose neurodegenerative diseases such as Korsakov, and other types of dementia, it cannot fathom a person's higher self. That core of the person exists at a deeper, protected, spiritual level: the level of the soul.

As we continue with Edward's narrative of living with Alzheimer's disease, I will argue, in parallel to Sacks' conclusion, that the soul is invulnerable even as the body decays. Just as the lotus flower retains the beauty of its pure white petals, even though it grows in swamps and murky rivers, so the soul is impervious to neurological devastation, however grave.

Thread of Awareness

In his book *The Mystic Heart,* Brother Wayne Teasdale defines awareness as the immortal nature of the mind. Connecting with awareness is the way we evolve into our true self. The method for this evolutionary transcendence is the *via negativa,* the process of elimination of what we are not. Teasdale says that when we see, and can eliminate from mind, those false ideas and opinions about ourselves that obscure our pure nature, then our divine inner buddha awakens. Mind and heart, understanding and compassion, join as our limited self – the ego – is transcended. We approach Christ consciousness – or, as it is called in the East, Self-realization. As Krishna tells Arjuna in the *Bhagavad Gita*: "He who is happy within his Self, and has found Its peace, and in whom the inner light shines, that sage attains Eternal Bliss and becomes Spirit Itself." [47] This desire to become one with Spirit remained strong in Edward even as his brain atrophied.

In Daniel Siegel's book, *Mind*, two modes of perception are described: the *bottom-up sensory conduit* and the *top-down constructor*. The bottom-up sensory conduit of perception uses the senses to draw into mind sense impressions in the present moment. Smelling, seeing, touching, hearing, tasting are bottom-up conduits of information and connection with the world around us. It could be argued that the senses are also messengers of intuition as we sometimes experience a sensitivity to our subtle surroundings through our senses. Non-locality also plays a part. When someone is staring at us from across a room, for example, we pick that energy up through the body. Sometimes, if the mind is quiet and attentive, we can intuit what is going on beneath the surface of observed behavior. As memory loss intensified, Edward relied more on the bottom-up conduit of perception. He was still able – perhaps more so than before – to sense the mood I was in as well as his own mood. As caregiver, I needed to be sensitive to his sensitivity.

Siegel argues that this bottom-up mode of

perception is underdeveloped in most of us. Often simple, sensory-based exchanges with our environment are missed because we are preoccupied with the second mode of perception, the top-down constructor mode. This mode is pre-baked with filters that are constructed out of prior experience. Learned beliefs and opinions stored in memory have precedence in how we view each moment, each event, and each person. Those opinions may not match in accuracy what is perceived. For example, we meet an acquaintance at a party and see the person, not with the fresh eyes of presence, but as we conceived him or her to be in the past. In the case of husband and wife, preconceived notions about each other are baked into the relationship over the years. These notions are difficult to uproot, much less see clearly. This challenge is compounded by the arrival of Alzheimer's disease. The relationship is destabilized; new information has entered it. Each day Edward and I were introduced to symptoms of this new element in our relationship. But this very destabilization can be seen as an opportunity for both spouses to recognize karmic flaws in the relationship and work to overcome them. In Eastern spirituality the word *karma* means *action*. Karma are habitual patterns of behavior, of action, that collect over lifetimes. These patterns can be positive or negative; that is, actions can promote spiritual evolution or impede it.

Using the top-down constructor mode to arrange our experiences in meaningful ways is necessary to forming a subjective self. However, as Siegel reminds us, being in the moment to receive and sift through the flow of new information which arouses sensations and feelings is just as important. Balance is needed between the two modes for the mind to function effectively in its task of integrating what is coming in with what is stored. If we stay present, we can oversee and discern what is valuable to retain and reject what awareness shows us to be false and inimical to spiritual growth. For optimum health, the two modes work together effectively when presence, or mindfulness, is the modus operandi.

The caregiver of the person living with Alzheimer's disease needs to understand these differing modes of perception for two reasons. First, the gradual loss of cognitive functions means that the ability to use learned experience degenerates in the person living with Alzheimer's disease. As the person ceases to be as he was, the caregiver must adjust and step in to provide cognitive help, without condescension. Secondly, even as neural connections in the temporal and frontal cortices of the brain begin to decay, the motor-sensory systems are still able to operate as bottom-up conduits. Understanding this shift, the caregiver can encourage the person living with Alzheimer's disease to reinforce his or her sensory connection to the world. For example, mindful walking out in the fresh air keeps the attention on the footfall; one feels the earth underneath and the space between steps. This connection to the present moment is the route whereby awareness is retained and exercised. In a later chapter we will consider how, as the constructor mode of perception falters in Alzheimer's patients, creative activities like drawing, performed in awareness and with imagination (a right hemisphere strength) can be bottom-up conduits that deliver meaning and joy.

When Edward gave his twenty-minute class in training the mind to stay in the Now, he was sensorily present. Long-term memories of the past emerged and fused with the present. His many years of tutoring classes in the subject he loved – Self-realization – came to the surface of his mind and impelled the thought-provoking dialogue he established with his niece's husband. Ego was not involved. It wasn't a planned lecture. Rather, it was an organic, spontaneous arising of truthful words that reflected Edward's lifelong investment in the study of spiritual knowledge. Imparting those words to others was an act of service.

Ironically, the present moment, though infiltrated by the past, is all any of us have. Edward had it absolutely in that brief but potent exchange. The cognitive gears in his brain were in full operation, guided by awareness which is timeless. When we are in the zone of this timelessness we are at the hub of choice and transformation.

Dr. Elizabeth Kübler-Ross, in her book *On Death and Dying*, states that it is never appropriate to treat the terminally ill patient as a vegetable simply because he or she cannot speak and does not respond to stimuli. She gives the example of a patient, Mrs. F., who had a debilitating disease compounded by a stroke. She could not speak. It was assumed by the hospital staff that her brain was no longer functioning. Mrs. F's daughter sat by her mother's side every day, silent and anxious about her mother's condition. When Kübler-Ross beckoned to the daughter to come with her so that, in conversation, the daughter might receive some support, Kübler-Ross looked back at the mother and spoke, saying that she would bring the daughter back shortly. The woman turned her head and looked at Kübler-Ross who immediately knew that the woman understood what she had just said. Her opinion of the woman's condition immediately changed. She realized that, even with Mrs. F's mental impairment, awareness was still behind the eyes of the woman. It was a lesson she would not forget.

In his study of the simple-minded, Oliver Sacks disputes the idea that the loss of abstract and conceptual thinking equates with mental regression. It is true that these people suffer from defective brain functions and are thereby limited to the world of the present moment. This loss, however, is not indicative of a descent into a sub-human state. Rather, Nature compensates for this loss by enhancing the gateway to sensibility and imagination, through what Sacks calls *the concrete*. Like Siegel's bottom-up conduit, the concrete is available through sensory awareness. Sacks affirms that even when the brain is damaged, a life with meaning is possible. For example, Rebecca, one of Sacks' patients, was physically handicapped and mentally defective. However, she loved going to synagogue; she knew all the chants. Rebecca never learned to read, but when she was in the natural world, which she loved, she would suddenly wax poetic about what she saw. Her ordinary movements were clumsy, but when she danced, she became graceful. Sacks' relationship with the simple-minded convinced him that reverting to the concrete is not regressive but a preservation by the brain of something essential to our personality and our humanity – something very close to our soul.

Journal Entries

In the following journal entries dated from 2019 to 2021 a thread of awareness can be seen in Edward's behavior. His awareness of cognitive decline occasionally peeks out like the sun from dense clouds. Sometimes this momentary realization of mental decline triggers a cover-up. Sometimes it bursts forth as lucidity – a sudden acknowledgement of the disease and the ability to speak about it as a detached spectator.

2019

8/14: We go to a concert at the retreat property of The School in Wallkill, NY. I am thinking it will make Edward happy to be back there, but a dark mood descends when we leave. As we drive home, he voices regret about leaving The School at age eighty, even though it was prompted by a decision to spend more time in Florida as we aged. I suggest that he can try going back to School in a way he can handle. The next morning, he remembers our conversation. He says, "how can I go back? I have Alzheimer's!" This is the first time he has acknowledged his condition. He quickly reverts to denial later in the day.

9/17: Edward goes shopping; he still drives. I give him an empty mayo jar and an ibuprofen bottle to match at the store. When he comes home I hear him in the garage shuffling around in the car. He comes in bewildered, not carrying the bag I gave him for the bought items. He says, "I remember buying the pills." I call Rite-Aid to see if he left the pill bottle there. They don't find anything. We go back into the garage to search. Finally, I see on the workbench the bag I had given him. The two items are inside. At dinner we speak about the incident. He is recognizing that his brain is not working normally. "What's happening to me?" he asks. "I have no recollection of walking around the car and putting the bag on the workbench. It's like a sudden switch, and then nothing. When I come out of it and catch myself, I am aware that time was lost. It's something that suddenly happens without my consent. Will this get worse?" I answer from my reading of how brain tissue deteriorates and causes haphazard and intermittent blanks at first. He asks more about Alzheimer's disease, showing some detachment. I am wondering if there is a way to consciously prevent further damage by mental focus, conscious attention. We talk about this. Wouldn't his physical exercises and meditation help? After the evening's meditation I ask him how it went. He says, "It was normal; I was attentive. But before, in those seconds in the garage, I have no memory of it."

10/5: Our friend Diane and her brother Robert visit us. Robert has an agile mind; he speaks quickly. Edward can't follow, stays quiet. I ask Edward to give Robert a tour of the house that he and our son John built. I hear him saying that his brother Ludge helped him build the house. When questioned on this by Diane he says, "I meant my son." But he asked me to take over the tour. I think he was aware of his mistake and afraid he'd make another slip.

2020

1/12: After supper I say there are cookies and ice cream for dessert. He says he'll have milk and a few cookies. I get these for him; he eats at the counter. Twenty minutes later he says, "I think I'll have some milk and cookies."

I say, "you already did."

He says, "Yes, I remembered that, but I'll have some more."

He's aware that he repeated himself and is covering up.

2/14-15: We're in Florida, beginning to pack up to sell

the condo. I ask Edward to pack up his tools that are on the pegboard in the garage. He doesn't want to. We argue. I don't handle it right because I begin putting his tools in a box. He demands I put all the tools back because he might need them. He says he will pack up next week. I argue that we need to pack incrementally. He sits for hours on the lanai brooding, almost catatonic. I should have let him do what he wanted to do. I finally apologize for pushing him.

The next day he puts all the tools back on the peg board. It's like Groundhog Day. I am angry. On my way to choir practice I shout, "Why did you do this? You need to cooperate; we're selling this place!"

"I didn't remember that," he says. I think he is using memory loss as an excuse to do what he wants.

The next morning, I see that he put the tools in the box after I went to sleep. He sleeps late, gets up in a bad mood. Before meditating he says angrily, "I'm dying!" This is the second time he has said this. Is he realizing that Alzheimer's is real and is damaging his brain? I feel so bad that I can't do anything about it.

After meditation he sees the Valentine's card and candy I left for him on the kitchen counter. He says, "I'm not all the good things the card says."

I say, "Yes you are."

Ludge calls and I hear Edward say, "I have Alzheimer's, like you." This is the first time I have heard Edward admit his condition out loud to anyone. He dries the dishes after lunch without being asked. He is making an effort to help out and get over his sour mood.

5/10: We sell the condo and are back in NY. We buy an electric lawn mower. I say to Edward, "let's work together on combining the parts." I take out the directions and ask him to read them out loud as we work. I see that he does not comprehend what he reads. He can't follow the directions.

To cover up and save face he says, "I'm just in the way. You take care of it." He goes upstairs. It hurts me to know that Edward is feeling humiliated and sidelined from life. His persona, so tied to his profession, is unable to perform and he knows it. I notice later that he is walking stiffly. His motor coordination may be affected.

He spills some wine on the carpet. "I spilt it because you are always watching me!" he shouts. He is aware that he is getting clumsy, but he covers it up by projecting blame onto me.

5/11: Edward can't follow the plot line of movies. At first, he blames it on the fast-paced style in contemporary movies. "Not like the old movies," he says. When I offer that maybe it is getting harder for him to follow the story, he queries, "maybe it's the Alzheimer's." His acknowledgement surprises me.

5/15: Edward gets very angry and starts crying when I push him to help me change the water softener filter. He doesn't remember that we had no trouble installing the filter last time. He insists through tears and rage that our son John should do it, that he can't and won't. He goes upstairs. I shouldn't have tried to convince him that it was easy if we worked together. I manage to change it by myself. Later, in trying to fortify the flower box where a screw had come loose, he gets upset until finally he is able to tighten the screw with the correct screwdriver. "Don't interfere," he yells, "this is what I do!" – referring to his profession. He is realizing that ordinary handyman tasks which used to be easy are challenging for him now. He also realizes that he is more dependent on me. This makes him angry. I must be careful not to push him. I must recognize his limits and his growing fragility as a man, both mentally and emotionally. I think his awkwardness embarrasses him and makes him think less of himself.

8/11: About fifteen minutes after we finish meditating, Edward asks if I am ready to meditate. This happens a lot. I say we already did. A few minutes later he asks again if we meditated, but this time with a little grin on his face. He is teasing me. He is aware that he hadn't been aware.

8/25: At lunch we have a high-level spiritual conversation. He speaks cogently about the effect of no longer being in The School which gave his life meaning. He goes on to reflect on what it was that allowed for this meaningful time in his life – forty-four years as a student and tutor. He says it was a certain "steadiness" related to purification and becoming "holy," even to a minimal degree. He says he once felt this but that it was missing now. "I feel rudderless," he says. "I'm going through daily motions but finding nothing meaningful." My heart aches as I listen to the intelligence and longing in his heart. I suggest that the meditation he does twice a day is an anchor, and spiritual study too, and he agrees, but he seems to want more – as he puts it, a "working connection to something higher than every day, ordinary stuff." This is a high-level thought process, well enunciated and differing from the frequent disconnections in his speech and actions due to Alzheimer's.

Earlier, for example, he was in the kitchen to pour more tea. The teapot was right in front of him, but he didn't see it. I had to point it out. It may not be his eyesight, but rather the eyes see the teapot, but the neural circuit that runs from the sensory perception to the visual cortex via optic nerves, and the resulting comprehension of what is seen, is fraying.

9/22: First day of fall. Edward sleeps longer. Today he sleeps until 11:00. I read that the sleep-waking cycle is regulated by the hypothalamus, deep within the medial temporal lobe, in communication with the brainstem. When I try to wake him, he says, "why should I get up? I have nothing meaningful to do." He says he thinks a lot about memories from his time in The School where he felt productive. "I'm in a dream most of the time," he says. This comment shows a witnessing of the disintegration process in his brain. At dinner he asks, "do you still have objectives in life? Because I don't." He is silent; then, "What day is it? How old am I?" The old questions repeat.

2021

1/22: More news about the looming impeachment trial of Trump and the insurrection. Edward asks again, "What impeachment? What insurrection?" I explain. "I don't remember anything about that," he says. "I wasn't paying attention." He is aware that he can't remember and uses the excuse of not paying attention to cover up for the shame he feels.

2/27: I ask him to shovel the snow on the back patio. I try to give him jobs to help him feel productive, in hopes that these tasks might stem the depression that can overtake him. He says my tone of voice is "curt"; he gets angry. I lose it and get angry too. After he shovels the snow he goes upstairs and lays down for a few hours. When he comes down for evening meditation, he apologizes.

"I'm sorry for all that," he says.

"Me too," I say. We hug.

A few hours had passed but he remembered the incident. Perhaps memory of an incident is retained when there is a strong emotional component to it. Edward's normal temperament is conciliatory and placid. When he sees his behavior as volatile and uncontrolled, it bothers him. He feels he is betraying the spiritual teaching which has given meaning to his life, particularly the practice of detachment and equanimity.

5/22: Sometimes he lies when he forgets or doesn't know how to do something. He is embarrassed, so lying is a defense. This manipulative behavior shows that the PFC is still intact, and awareness is operating. On Sunday evenings he always watches *60 Minutes*. I tell him to go upstairs while I finish cleaning up the dinner dishes, press the TV on-button, and then press channel 2 on the remote. When I call, "Do you have the program on?" he says, "Yes."

When I go up to join him, he is not watching *60 Minutes*. He dissembles, saying he was watching it, but it was over, and he was watching something else. I switch to channel 2; *60 Minutes* is still on. I should not give him a sequence of actions he is not able to do.

6/12: Two items in the news on TV: Biden's visit to the G7 meeting in London and the Wimbledon tennis tournament. Edward mixes them up. When I say that Biden is going to visit the queen he responds, "Did he win the tournament?" Then realizing his gaffe, he laughs, and so do I. Awareness, which is still there, is the backdrop to the gaffe and the realization of the gaffe.

11/13: This evening Edward is energized and lucid. It is an awakening that reminds me of the male patient in the film *Awakenings*, who for a brief time returns to normal. We are in the bedroom getting ready to go to sleep when he suddenly begins talking, his face and gestures lit with joy. He is suddenly aware of his condition and becomes euphoric.

"I was totally unaware that I was in decline," he begins, "but now I know it. I'm now aware of it as I haven't been in the past." His voice rises with excitement.

"How did the awareness arise?" I ask.

"My head usually feels fuzzy," he says. "but today is totally different! Now I know I have Alzheimer's. This admission is a big step down. It feels disabling. Before, I felt normal, even though I wasn't."

"Awareness, realization of this condition, is a positive thing," I say. "Don't let it be a step down."

"There's something very amazing about this," he says, laughing, as if he is high. "Why haven't I recognized this earlier? Yet other people knew it. I'm dependent now, no one depends on me now. I have an awakening today, a rude awakening. This is like a grace. What's happening is happening; it is what it is. If I get up and take three steps to the window that's what happens, simple. Today is different, an awakening. It exploded and others knew it and I didn't know it. I'm still intelligent enough to say, 'so be it'; no need to pretend or cover it."

He pauses for a moment, considering his next words. "I hope I perish before I need help. I want to be my own person. This is the first day of knowing death is at my doorstep. Easy come, easy go. It's going to be different now. Before it was hid. Now it's in the open."

11/21: Edward seems to have forgotten his 'awakening' of eight days ago. He resumes the repeated questions like "Where do I sleep? Do I sleep with you? Which side of the bed? How old am I?" He remains anxious a lot of the time and disoriented. A wave of dread washes over me as we sit on the sofa, snuggling.

12/26: We go to James' house to celebrate his son Jonah's sixteenth birthday. We sing Happy Birthday and then Edward says, "aren't we going to sing Happy Birthday?" Everyone gets quiet.

I murmur, "we already did."

"A second time," he says, smiling. We all laugh to ease the moment of unease.

That Edward could respond quickly to correct his error showed awareness and creativity.

**

The oldest part of the human brain, the brainstem, contains the medulla. One of the functions of the medulla is to arouse the brain and body to alertness by regulating levels of consciousness or awareness. Being awake is being aware. The youngest part of the brain, the prefrontal cortex (PFC), has a more complex role in enabling awareness.

Fundamental to the executive functions that the PFC performs, including working memory and self-awareness, is the primary energy of awareness. So, both the oldest and youngest areas of the brain control levels of consciousness or awareness in the body. This fact prompts the question: is there a fundamental level of consciousness which dwells in all life forms? When Arjuna asks Krishna in the *Bhagavad Gita,* "Who are you?" Krishna replies, "I am the Self, seated in the hearts of all beings; I am the beginning and the life, and I am the end of them all." [48] Self or Spirit is the source of consciousness that resides in all beings. The brain of the human being is arguably the most complex, but also the most non-specialized neurological structure in the evolutionary development of life forms. This non-specialization opens doors of possibilities for creative evolutionary growth, possibilities that stem from the capacity of the human being to be consciously aware of awareness. Yet all beings, including us, are living by the grace of consciousness. Each has its own special gift to offer to life. The flower has its color and scent, the butterfly its dainty wings, the bear its strength. One could go on and on.

In a story that recounts a conversation between Buddha and one of his disciples, Buddha teaches the primacy of awareness – of just being – as the way to enlightenment.

Disciple: Who are you? Are you a guru?

Buddha: No.

Disciple: Are you a wizard? Or a shaman?

Buddha: No.

Disciple (getting frustrated): Are you an avatar?

Buddha: No.

Disciple: So what are you?

Buddha: I am awake!

A thread of awareness underlies the loss of short-term memory, even as the latter confines the person living with Alzheimer's disease to the present tense. Sparks of awareness will continue to provide the light of sanity, but as the disease advances, new, sometimes disturbing, signs will show themselves. We consider these continuing signs of Alzheimer's disease in the next chapter.

Chapter Four: **Continuing Signs**

Along with short-term memory loss there are progressive symptoms of cognitive decline that, over time, become more prevalent and observable as areas of the cerebral cortex atrophy. These progressive symptoms include forgetting not just what happened a moment ago but forgetting more permanent things like who friends and even family members are. "Who is that man in the living room?" Edward asked when his niece and her husband visited at Christmas, 2022. Longstanding daily routines became harder for Edward to remember as a sequence of events. His morning routine had always been exercising, showering, dressing, meditating, and then having tea while sitting in the wing-back chair and reading the newspaper. Now he came to the kitchen in his exercise pants to have tea, forgetting the intervening activities. Following a routine is easy; in fact, it often happens on automatic pilot. We may be absent-minded, in and out of awareness, yet we are still able to carry out sequential actions. But for persons living with Alzheimer's disease, routine becomes a challenge as the neural connections between the hippocampus – the central memory hub – and the planning/deciding faculty of the PFC become clogged with beta-amyloid plaque and tau tangles.

Edward's ability to comprehend what he read in the newspaper became spotty at best. "What is Covid?" he asked after we had been reading about it, living with it, and wearing masks for a year. He was forgetting where objects were in space. He couldn't summon an image in his mind of the layout of rooms in the house or how to navigate from one room to another. Navigation depends on a functioning hippocampus. Edward would lose the sense of where his body was in space. This ability is regulated by the proprioceptive function of the parietal lobe. Common questions were "where do I sleep tonight?" or "Where is the garage?" When he began to forget to take his Memantine medication twice daily I began to oversee this important part of his routine. I was now paying the bills and doing the taxes. Driving became hazardous for Edward. He couldn't discern where the road met the shoulder. He forgot common routes like driving to and from the supermarket.

This loss of connection to the outer environment was compounded by Edward's visual impairment of macular degeneration and his hearing loss. It made him angry when the eye doctor advised that he stop driving. He saw his world shrinking. He would intertwine a news story with a call I was making to the doctor; he would mix up discrete actions as if they were related. The ability to recognize and distinguish objects – the task of the inferotemporal cortex (IT) – also began to fail. The operation of the IT is overseen by the PFC which gets involved in recognition of stimuli when they are ambiguous. One day, in picking up a clementine for a snack, Edward said "do I peel it?" which meant "do I eat the peel too?"

Perhaps the hardest thing to witness, as his caregiver, was Edward's reaction to the loss of faculties associated with his sense of identity, even his masculinity. He became frustrated when he couldn't do simple things like making a fire. He felt himself becoming more vulnerable and isolated – a prisoner in his own home, unable, as he often said, to go anywhere because he couldn't drive. Not being able to drive, not comprehending what he read in the newspaper or saw on TV, alarmed him. The well-worn pages of his spiritual books were now a challenge to his ability to understand the words that once nourished his mind. All this attenuation of his ego and his mind was devastating to him – and to me. I watched an uptick in emotional instability and anxiety when his ability to control emotional outbursts deteriorated. Edward was experiencing mood swings from passivity to anger to depression that were foreign to his usual even temperament. His sensitivity to perceived slights and his defensive behavior, though known to me during our marriage as times for me to back off, increased. Because the person living with Alzheimer's disease is losing his ability to control his emotions, it is up to the caregiver to help the loved one by understanding and defusing these mood swings.

A familiar psychological pattern of feeling abandoned and deprived was surfacing in Edward's behavior. This feeling of deprivation never made sense to me because his mother was the epitome of a loving parent. However, Edward did not have a good relationship with his father who was schooled in the traditional, chauvinistic upbringing of Eastern European culture. In immigrating to America in the 1920s, his father carried this tradition with him. Edward saw the fights that broke out between his parents. Several times he watched his father beat his mother; he sided with his mother. He married me, a strong-willed woman like his mother. The marital arguments that we had often flared up over his felt sense that I was criticizing him.

Old, hidden feelings and vulnerabilities can resurface in

Alzheimer's disease. A friend of ours, Inga, who developed Alzheimer's in her eighties, was described by her caregiver as displaying a feisty, angry temperament as the disease progressed. Previously known for her aloof calm, the sudden eruption of anger and resentment surprised the caregiver. In her book *On Death and Dying*, Kübler-Ross tells the story of a young nun who was hospitalized eleven times with Hodgkins' disease. She displayed a lot of anger, so much so that the nurses and other hospital staff avoided her. Their resentment of her behavior resulted in her receiving less care than she needed. When called in by the hospital chaplain, Kübler-Ross began a dialogue with the nun to discover the cause of her persistent anger. The nun's story revealed a deep-seated resentment of her mother who required that she fit the pattern of womanhood by learning how to embroider and do other feminine activities like her sisters. The nun was gregarious, an extrovert, more like her father. Cooped up in the house she felt like an outsider, the black sheep of her large family. At age thirteen, she decided to repress her own identity and become a nun to please her mother. She took vows at age twenty. She contracted Hodgkin's disease at age forty-one. During the first interview, Kübler-Ross allowed the nun to vent her feelings – her anger – without interference or judgment. As the visits continued, the nun felt more comfortable in Kübler-Ross's presence. She unloaded the story of her childhood, her unmet needs. The conversations were like a confession that liberated the nun from acting out her unresolved issues. Her behavior began to change. A natural warmth surfaced. This thawing in her personality drew an equivalent solicitude from the hospital staff. Unburdened, she left the hospital, cheerful and relieved that the mental-emotional pain she had lived with had vanished. She died at home shortly after leaving the hospital.

When Edward became anxious or angry, I tried to ease his emotional pain by hugs and words of comfort. I reminded him, and myself, that he was more than his body and mind. Nevertheless, bouts of depression would seize him, and he would sit stone-faced and glum until they passed. There were also moments of frivolity and lightness which showed that a sense of humor was still available to him. Once, when I was cleaning the cat pan, Edward objected, saying, "that's my job; we have a union around here." And when I began giving him piano lessons he would joke about his "prowess" at the piano.

Edward began to sleep longer hours in the morning. During the day he dozed off while sitting on the sofa listening to soothing music. We still went out shopping together. He pushed the cart to exercise his legs, but after walking up and down several aisles he said he needed to sit down; he was tired. According to an article in the New York Times *Science Times*, research shows that brisk walking after age eighty keeps the brain healthy and can lessen the impact of Alzheimer's disease.[49] Edward was never a walker; nor did he embrace cardiac exercise. I convinced him to walk with me daily around the block, but the distance covered got shorter and shorter as he complained of fatigue and stiffness in his legs. His balance became uncertain. I would hold his arm to steady him, wondering if the motor cortex in his brain was atrophying.

Journal entries

The following journal entries from 2019 to 2022 chart some of the progressive signs described above. They bring to life the ongoing chronology of our experience with Alzheimer's disease. Advanced signs occasionally appeared early in the presentation of the disease. Later, these advanced signs developed into more chronic behavior.

2019

9/18: Today was difficult. I fractured my left ankle two weeks ago and I am in a boot. Edward drives me to SUNY to give the class I am teaching. We agree he will pick me up. Meanwhile he will wait at the café, enjoying a latte. He forgets the sequence. As he drives home the car hits a deer. He goes to the body shop for an estimate. He tells me later that he didn't see the deer. I wonder if his loss of peripheral vision is involved. I wait at the college for one and a half hours for him to return. I call him but he doesn't pick up. He forgets where I am. I call James' wife, Ronnie, and she comes to pick me up. When I arrive home he is sitting on the wing-back chair, mystified as to where I was. We must go to the eye doctor. He shouldn't be driving. I know he will resist because the idea of driving is associated with freedom, independence, and masculinity.

10/2: When I ask Edward in the evening to put the cat bowls in the sink, fill them with soapy water, and leave them to soak, he fills them with water and puts them back on the cats' tray on the floor. The combination of small tasks is complex for him. His inability to follow the sequence shows a confusion in hearing, remembering, organizing, and executing several instructions. I am reading that several areas of the brain, like the auditory area in the temporal lobe, the hippocampus, and the prefrontal cortex, need to work together in sequenced actions. What I asked him to do was too much for him. But if I stay with him and coach him through a sequence, he gets angry. He has difficulty remembering how the toaster oven works. I draw a big diagram with a black marker and tape it to the wall behind the toaster oven, but it doesn't help. He still can't press the right buttons. We laugh about it, and he says later "I f*cked up." He gets down on himself for these lapses; he feels humiliated.

2020

4/16: For about a week Edward has missed the routine evacuation of his bowels. It was a morning regularity, like clockwork. Is this a new sign? Last night he got up in the middle of the night to poop. I asked him in the morning if it was so urgent that he needed to go. He said no; nothing came out. Bowel irregularities are symptomatic of chronic neurological diseases like Parkinson's and Alzheimer's. Both urination and defecation are eliminative processes controlled by the autonomic nervous system. I read that usually urinary incontinence precedes bowel incontinence.

4/18: We garden together. I give him one simple task and he can do it. I avoid a task with several parts, such as "carry pine bark nuggets to the area, dump, and then spread them." When we finish and come inside, we wash our hands in the basement sink, then go upstairs. He begins washing his hands in the kitchen sink. I ask him why he is doing that since we had just washed them in the basement. He says he didn't remember. We laugh about it, and I refer to Lady Macbeth which triggers another laughing bout. I realize he is totally in the present tense but a few seconds later that 'present' is past and forgotten.

5/11: When I get two plates out for dessert, I see that

one has crumbs of bread on it from his lunch. He put some dishes away without washing them.

5/25: At dinner I ask him "how did you like the risotto for lunch?"

He replies, "did I have lunch?"

When we go upstairs to watch the news, I hand him the earphones because of his hearing loss; he doesn't seem to recognize them. Once I tell him what they are, he asks me if I want to use them.

6/6: Edward put a pair of trousers, rolled up, in a drawer with his short sleeve shirts. We finally find them after a lengthy search.

8/25: After evening meditation we talk about his bladder medication. I say, "the doctor prescribed it."

He responds, "we meditated for half an hour."

His brain was stuck, fixated in one concept and unable to discern the change in subject. This is a first. It may have to do with meditation being important to him, so he falls back to speaking about that when he loses the thread of a conversation.

9/15: He says at dinner, "I feel strange – like I don't know where I am, though I know where I am." He is trying to define the feeling. "I feel placeless, homeless." He pauses, then asks, "do you believe in successive lives?"

12/2: For the second day Edward asks me, "are you satisfied with your life?" He is still able to think philosophically about himself. The PFC is still operating. When I turn the question to him, he hesitates. He says the best part was School but "I could have done more with my life." He spends much of the afternoon bringing his brush painting materials upstairs from the garage and organizing them. It seems illogical since he would practice his art in the garage. I had offered to help him set up a place on the workbench. This flurry of activity may be an effort to feel like he's doing something worthwhile.

12/8: Edward meshes two news stories together – a previous story about Trump's border wall and a eulogy for a Covid victim.

2021

1/8: Around 9:00 pm, after I get Edward's pajamas out for him and bring them to the TV room, he asks, "where do I sleep?"

Astounded, but trying not to show alarm, I say "in our bedroom," pointing in that direction.

"Let me see." he says, getting up from the couch and coming with me to the hall. We walk to the bedroom. He then recognizes the room.

Edward often says, "I feel lost." This is a feeling of despair, but it is also literal, losing a sense of physical orientation. He is increasingly unable to hold in mind a map of the house where we have lived for eleven years.

1/10: Lots of TV news about the storming of the Capitol. Edward inserts a comment about football as if it was related, then realizes his mistake – he is aware of it – and laughs.

1/16: Edward still has a sense of humor. He comes down to the garage to help me clean the car. I ask him what he was doing upstairs.

He said, "meditating."

I said, "but we already did."

He joked, "right, I must have needed it."

2/10: I need to go over to James' house to dog-sit most of the day. Edward doesn't want to come so I prepare his lunch before I leave. When I get home, I see that he forgot the prepared lunch and ate something else. He had dumped the contents of the kitchen garbage can into the recycling container. He also left the downstairs bathroom faucet running which really upset me. Did he not hear the water running? Did he just forget to turn the water off? I scold him, but I apologize later. He can't help it. We don't talk much after dinner. He is quiet and seems depressed. I notice now that when he forgets, or does something inappropriate, he gets frustrated and reacts in three possible ways: 1) deflects and laughs it off to cover up; 2) becomes meek, submissive, and quiet (stews); or 3) projects, giving me dagger eyes and angry words as if it is my fault. I mustn't take the bait but try to remain positive, detached, but also loving. I must put the teaching into practice; stay present with him. Sometimes this is hard, tiring, and makes me sad.

3/16-4/1: We are on a two-week Florida vacation, staying in a rental house two blocks from Indian Rocks Beach. He will be able to walk the distance easily. But it is now obvious that any change in venue confuses him and heightens the disorientation that he feels even at home. The vacation is of little interest to him. He asks if his mother is coming down to visit.

"Who?" I ask, surprised.

"My mother, Mum."

"She passed away years ago," I say. I see recognition in his eyes. He is mystified as to why he said this. But he asks about his mother again, numerous times. In this strange place, is he looking for the childhood comfort and security associated with his mother?

6/25: He can't tell the difference between our two cats: Simon, a white half-Siamese cat, and Henry, an orange tabby cat. Is this confusion due to neurological damage in the inferotemporal cortex (IT) that regulates the recognition of objects?

12/14: Another sudden mood swing – active amygdala. The day started off fine as Edward awoke in a good mood, but it drastically changed. After exercising and before showering (he was keeping to his routine so far), I come into the bathroom to make sure I put fresh underwear where he can see it. He says, "Get the f*ck out of here! I'm sick and tired of you!" Cursing is so uncharacteristic of Edward. I feel hurt but I must remember that these outbursts are the disease, not him.

Later, on the way to James' law office (he is going to have lunch with his son while I have a much needed reiki treatment) he says, "I'm in a bad mood." He is aware of how he feels.

"Maybe lunch with your son will lift the mood," I say. When I see him later he is himself again, the morning's despondency gone.

12/24: The chimney sweep man comes to give an

estimate on repair. Edward gets nasty, calls him a crook when he hears the price. Pre-Alzheimer's Edward would be able to control his feelings. He would react reasonably to the cost of repair. But the disease dispenses with filters. The amygdala, which is primed to react to threats, is engaged. The prefrontal cortex is not able to act like a brake to restrain what comes out of his mouth.

2022

4/17: Easter Day. I bake a coconut cake. We have a piece for dessert, then the Easter candies I bought for Edward. He loves chocolate. When he finishes the candies, he asks if we are going to have cake too. I offer to turn on the TV. He scoffs and says, "do you think I can't do it?!"

***

Denial, Delusion, Depression – the three Ds

As the symptoms of Alzheimer's disease accelerated in frequency, Edward displayed three mental-emotional states that signaled a more dramatic loss of synaptic neural connections. These three states were denial (mixed with anger), delusion, and depression. As Edward's outbursts of anger intensified, the shielding power of denial weakened. I wondered if both the hippocampus and the prefrontal cortex were losing their ability to inhibit the amygdala's unbridled readiness to react according to the fight-or-flight reflex. I began to be on guard, as there was no way to know when he would lose his composure or what would trigger an outburst.

The frequent overlapping of denial, delusion, and depression added fuel to the intensity of each of the three mental-emotional states. A leap to a more advanced stage of the disease was occurring. Even so, Edward's awareness of what was happening was still visible, like sparks of light in the dark – fireworks at times.

Denial

How we respond to a health crisis can be an opportunity for spiritual growth. To acknowledge and accept the physical fact that wayward proteins are killing the source of thought and feeling – one's brain – is a hard thing to do. The belief that 'I am not this sickness; I am not this body' is a deep spiritual truth which can summon forth the courage to face such a grave diagnosis. Edward had read the great teachers, like Nisargadatta and Shankara. He believed their pronouncement that 'I am not this body; I am the imperishable Self.' He liked to recite Shakespeare's *Sonnet 146,* which in part reads:

Poor soul, the centre of my sinful earth, ...

Within be fed, without be rich no more.

So shalt thou feed on Death, that feeds on men.

And Death once dead, there's no more dying then.[50]

Nevertheless, Edward vacillated in confronting the fact that he had Alzheimer's disease. Mostly in denial mode, he had occasional bursts of recognition of his condition, but these admissions were quickly covered over with denial. He was not able to fully accept the disintegration of his brain until late in the progression of the disease. It is one thing to know the truth intellectually, even spiritually, but facing your own imminent death brings into play the strong connection we all have to the body which is the material definition of our identity.

In her study of the terminally ill, Kübler-Ross broke through the taboo that surrounds talking about death and dying. Her discoveries inspired the rise of the Hospice movement. In interviews with patients, she discovered that there are universal stages in the process of dying. She labeled these progressive stages denial, anger, bargaining, depression, and acceptance. She found that people do not go through the stages in a uniform way. Rather, the stages are porous; they can intersect and overlap. Moreover, they are experienced in ways suited to the individual's history and needs. I would add that *sanskaric patterns* may play a role in how a person receives news of a terminal illness and deals with it. *Sanskara* is the Sanskrit word for the thread of *karma* (actions) that accumulate over successive lifetimes. In Hinduism and Buddhism, reincarnation is believed to be the vehicle by which we can evolve if we direct our lives to recognizing and overcoming psychological impediments through spiritual practice. Because the brain is the organ that differentiates the stages of the dying process, it may be that those stages blur in cases of dementia, especially in the advanced stage when the disease spreads to the prefrontal cortex. However, awareness is still operating, so at some level the stages play out.

The first stage, denial, can occur off and on throughout the months and years of a terminal illness. The persistence of denial was true in Edward's experience. When David's wife, Karen, developed early-onset Alzheimer's disease in 2014, at age sixty-three, the signs appeared in ways that were not dramatic at first, particularly because she had suffered a severe case of Lyme's disease which can affect the neurological system. Karen also developed sleep apnea. Research is showing a connection between prolonged, severe sleep apnea and the risk of developing Alzheimer's disease. For four years this disease festered, virtually unseen. During this time, she developed spinal stenosis and underwent successful surgery. David hoped the surgery would eliminate the brain fog that both he and Karen were noticing in her behavior. She used to love to read; she had stopped reading. She couldn't follow the story line in movies or do crossword puzzles anymore. She would get sleepy in the early evening. When short-term memory loss affected her thriving psychotherapy practice, it was clear to both David and Karen that something was wrong. The official diagnosis came in 2018. Karen did not at first deny she had Alzheimer's disease. She openly talked about it. As the knowledge of her condition sank in, she became afraid. Denial and anger set in. She was incensed that a person with her intellectual abilities could have Alzheimer's disease. The stew of emotions she was experiencing intensified for the next three years, along with depression. She lashed out verbally at her husband who became an ambivalent figure in her life – as David puts it, "I was her savior and her enemy at the same time."

Michael's wife, Eileen, reacted to her diagnosis in 2010 with shame. She had a visceral reaction to the stigma associated with Alzheimer's disease. Denial was deflected to others; she didn't want anyone else but her husband to know. When Eileen overheard Michael tell a good friend over the phone that his wife had Alzheimer's disease she was enraged. He promised he wouldn't tell anybody else without her permission. As an employee for twenty years in the management office of a prestigious apartment complex on Central Park West in New York City, Eileen was reliable, well-organized, and respected. When she began to misplace items, leave files unattended in piles on her desk, and make mistakes on mathematical calculations, she became sad and ashamed. She saw her intelligence slipping away. She suspected dementia. Her co-workers loved her and kindly gave her a farewell party. Michael told me it was hard to watch her try to do normal things like making a salad; she couldn't even cut an avocado. He said she was loved by many and showed love to many, including himself. Their bond was close. She often told her husband that she felt humiliated and wanted to die. With his quick wit Michael would rejoin, "Ok, let's go to the George Washington Bridge so you can jump off!"

Four years into the illness, Eileen went into what Michael calls "a hostility period" when anger would interlace with shame. "I knew this wasn't her. The loss of capacities hurt her so much that she had to unload the rage. People with Alzheimer's have to express this toxicity."

According to Kübler-Ross, denial, based in fear, is often a necessary cushion to allow the mind time to process what is happening to the body. Through processing the fact of the body's terminal condition, the patient will more easily arrive at acceptance. He or she will be willing to let go of this life. The caregiver must allow this buffer of denial and anger to play itself out, while attending with loving care and respect to the needs of the afflicted person. Edward's denial was mixed with anger as the disease progressed. As his caregiver, I had to learn not to take his spiteful words personally but allow the anger to be expressed. I hoped that, through expressing his feelings, Edward would reach acceptance.

Empathy will be the caregiver's natural response, says Kübler-Ross, if, in those times of friction in the relationship, she faces the fears that may surround her own terminal existence. Kübler-Ross contends that the journey towards death will be easier for the patient if those in the helping professions, like nurses and chaplains, listen to their patients. It is the patients who are their teachers. The nurse or chaplain can then help family members to be in tune with where the patient is in the dying process and give the appropriate support.

It may be helpful to review what happens physiologically when one is faced with a traumatic event – in this case, finding out one has a terminal illness. Fear and anger are aroused. This arousal is followed by an underlying anxiety which may be accompanied by projection of blame onto another person, usually the caregiver. In *Buddha's Brain*, authors Hanson and Mendius detail the sequence of physical reactions that developed in human history as an evolutionary adaptation to the threat of predators. Survival depended upon constant vigilance and a quick reaction to events – the fight-or-flight reflex. When fear or anger is aroused by a perceived threat, the sympathetic nervous system responds through the limbic and endocrine systems. The amygdala sounds the alarm; the thalamus relays danger to the brainstem which releases norepinephrine into the brain while the hypothalamus sends a signal to the pituitary gland to release stress hormones via the adrenal glands. Adrenaline and cortisol flood the body.[51] These hormones suppress the hippocampus which usually controls and inhibits the amygdala along with the PFC. The negativity bias in the brain intensifies feelings of fear and/or anger. Continually living in this stressful *red zone* is not healthy. Siegel, in his book *Mind*, notes that the release of cortisol due to severe stress adversely affects the hippocampus. In Alzheimer's disease, the hippocampus is one of the first parts of the brain to be affected. Siegel poses the question as to whether an excessive secretion of cortisol due to a traumatic event might put the hippocampus out of commission temporarily, and even severely damage it.

Journal entries

The following journal entries are selected to show Edward's use of denial and anger as a defense mechanism. While acknowledging Kübler-Ross's advice that people living with a terminal illness need time to adjust to their situation by passing through the stages of denial and anger, it is also important that the caregiver try to balance this venting process with activities that calm the person. Such calming activities can prevent the physical reactions described above from getting out of control. Providing soothing energy to reduce the temperature of agitation may involve just sitting with the loved one and holding his hand, listening to quiet music, going on a nature walk, or meditating together. Sometimes the right words of comfort and empathy arise in times of silent companionship. As the poet Rumi writes: "Now be silent. / Let the One who creates the words speak. / He made the door, / He made the lock, / He also made the key." [52]

2019

7/25: Again, the hearing aids battle. Sitting on the porch, a beautiful sunny day. "Hearing stimulates the brain," I say, "connecting the senses to sense objects through attention; you know, the Teaching 101, being present."

"I am present," he says. A wren is singing.

"Can you hear that?" I ask.

"No," he says.

"It's a wren, a beautiful song," I say. He can't hear high registers, including his cell phone ring.

"I can hear well enough. I don't need to hear the bird," he says. "I can hear you and I'm rarely in social gatherings."

"But you are missing out and it's important to stimulate the brain when you have Alzheimer's," I say. Mistake. He gets angry.

"I feel fine! Maybe I should just pack up and move out!" he shouts.

2020

5/31: Edward gets tired now after exerting even a modicum of energy. Even standing while drying dishes tires him. He's more sedentary and often complains of being cold and needing an extra jacket. It's hard to get him to go out for a walk. He spends most of the day sitting on the porch with the newspaper or his spiritual study material on his lap. Often, he just sits listless, apathetic. He says his life is a blank. When I ask him what he read he can't remember. Or he may fabricate events that aren't happening like "there's a war in Europe right now." When we speak about aging – and Alzheimer's – he doesn't like to talk about it, or he equivocates, saying "the doctor said I have eight to ten years before it hits."

"No," I say, "that's not what he said."

I begin to explain but he ignores my response and, in denial mode, says, "I don't feel any different than I ever did. I just stay in the present and that's all I can do" – an astute comment, even though it may not be the result of practice at this point, but of short-term memory loss.

12/8: Today is tough. When I come home from Tuesday morning shopping I see that Edward has not followed his morning routine. If I'm not here the routine doesn't happen. I ask him to snake the blocked kitchen sink. He tries but gets frustrated and angry. We argue. After he goes upstairs to shower, he sits in the bedroom stone-faced and unresponsive. I go upstairs and initiate a conversation about his negativity.

He shouts, "I'm dying! I can't do these things anymore. I'm a victim."

I say, "No, you have a choice of attitude."

But he is in the darkness. I leave the room.

Later he comes out of the dark mood but the anger and anxiety of losing his independence, his agency – his mind – is always there behind the event of the moment. I feel powerless to help him.

2021

1/11: Edward keeps coming in from the TV room to get his pajamas and I keep telling him to change in here when he is ready to go to sleep. I am reading in bed. It's 9:00 and Edward is confused and tired – sundown syndrome. He comes into the bedroom once again, aggrieved and cursing. It's like being hit.

He says angrily, "I sleep there," pointing to where I am, and I say, "no, you sleep on the other side."

He yells, "you treat me like sh*t!" He picks up Simon,

who had jumped off the bed, frightened by Edward's tone of voice. He throws him back on the bed. "And here's your f*cking cat!"

I don't react but inside I'm trembling. I take two Tylenol and one melatonin pill, but sleep is long in coming.

6/28: When Edward comes down in his exercise pants, I see he isn't wearing underwear. I ask him to go back to the bedroom and put some on. He blows up. I am silent. He goes out to the porch to meditate, then comes back in, crying. I sit down across from him.

"What's wrong with me?" he says, then, "you know I'd never harm you."

"Of course you wouldn't," I say. "It's Alzheimer's, not you."

"I don't want to hear that," he says, his voice quivering.

"I know, but it's the truth. It's not you," I reply. He doesn't answer. "Can I come over and sit with you?" I ask.

He nods. I sit close. I tell him I love him.

"Is this the beginning of something or the end?" he asks.

"I don't know," I say. I sense his fear.

"How can you even want to touch me?" he says.

"We don't touch enough," I say. He tears up.

After a few minutes he gets up and, turning to me, says, "I guess the best thing I can do right now is meditate."

1/14: Edward is becoming compulsively repetitive, asking the old questions like "where do I sleep? Are we married? How old am I?". I feel his anxiety, his desire to hold on to sanity. He mistakes the landline phone for the TV remote and tries to turn off the TV with it.

Today he asks, "are we living in Manhattan or the Bronx?"

"We live in Gardiner, in the Hudson Valley," I say. When he makes these 'mistakes' I know he knows the cause, so he gets defensive and angry.

At dinner he asks, "why would we come up to NY to just go back down?"

"Where do you think we are?" I ask.

"Florida," he says.

"How can that be?" I say, pointing to the window. "Look at the snow outside." He gets angry.

He says, "it pisses me off when you get angry!"

"I'm not angry," I say, "you are."

He's projecting his own anger onto me. He is suffering.

***

Delusion

Anecdotal evidence shows a proclivity in persons with Alzheimer's disease to go into an imaginary world of ideas, acted out in abnormal behavior. Psychotic symptoms such as delusions, hallucinations, and even paranoia appear later in the progression of the disease. They can, however, appear at an earlier stage, along with agitation, anxiety, mood swings, and loss of motivation or apathy. In people with Alzheimer's disease, and other dementias, the estimate of how prevalent neuropsychiatric symptoms (NPS) are runs as high as 97 per cent.[53] Safe and reliable pharmaceutical treatments are still being researched. Some anti-psychotic drugs can have serious side effects. Currently, the anti-psychotic drug Aripiprazole appears to give the best balance of effectiveness and safety for dementia psychosis.

Delusions and hallucinations can occur together, exposing a belief in an alternate reality, but they are not the same. Delusions are false beliefs, whereas hallucinations are imaginary sensory perceptions – usually auditory and/or visual. Hallucinations can involve several brain areas including the primary auditory cortex and language areas, sensory cortex, insula, hippocampus, inferior parietal lobe, and occipital lobe where the visual cortex is located.

Common delusions affecting people with Alzheimer's disease are persecutory delusions, such as suspicion of theft, infidelity, and abandonment. In the last twelve months of Karen's life, her delusional words and actions became more violent and accusatory. While David tried to maintain his composure she would insult him, saying things like "you're just a deadbeat; it's my money you want." He knew she couldn't help herself, but he also knew that he needed support. He turned to a friend who came and stayed with Karen occasionally so he could go out. David also attended some Alzheimer's Association meetings. When people with Alzheimer's disease believe dead people to be alive, it may not be as easy for the caregiver to distinguish between delusion and forgetfulness due to hippocampal damage. Edward's belief that I stole his wallet was a persecutory delusion. His references to his mother and brother as still alive could either be delusionary or a consequence of memory loss.

Misidentification syndromes can signal more serious cognitive and perceptual impairment. They present a challenge to the caregiver. These misidentifications may include the belief that a stranger is living in one's home (phantom boarder syndrome) or that loved ones – especially one's spouse – are impostors. Images on TV are believed to be real and the person one sees in the mirror is a stranger. In their presentation, these behaviors that occur in Alzheimer's disease have marked similarities to those in people suffering from schizophrenia. It is proposed by scientists that genetic predispositions to both schizophrenia and Alzheimer's disease are present in Alzheimer's psychosis.

In 1923, Jean Marie Joseph Capgras, a French psychiatrist, and his colleague Jean Reboul-Lachaux, published a paper that recounted evidence of what they called *illusion of doubles*. They proposed that a disconnect between the emotional and cognitive recognition of a face, due to brain damage, created an agnosia of identification. Agnosia is a neurological disorder in which a person is unable to recognize and name objects, persons, or even sounds. Their theory turned out to be correct and applicable to dementias such as Alzheimer's disease.

This inability to recognize a familiar face or object became known as the Capgras delusion. Modern studies of the Capgras delusion have located a marker in the skin conductance response (SRC) that shows a deficit in the autonomic nervous system. This system should trigger recognition of a familiar face. To the person living with Alzheimer's disease, the person being seen – such as his spouse – looks like someone he knows, but she must be an imposter. In Edward's case, the Capgras delusion was activated as the disease progressed. This will be shown in the journal entries below. In another type of delusion, called the Frégoli delusion, strangers are believed to be relatives or old friends from one's past. Edward experienced this delusion as early as the first year of his diagnosis.

Imagination is a central part of the creative process that any inventor, artist, or master chef depends on for inspiration. The right hemisphere of the brain, particularly the right prefrontal cortex, is associated with the creative process. Also involved is the limbic system, particularly the hippocampus and amygdala. It is interesting that these areas of creativity are also the areas of false beliefs and behaviors. When the imagination is used to form ideas that are stubbornly held as real, then the brain is concocting a distorted vision of reality. As Alzheimer's disease progresses, it appears that the elemental sense of self, as well as the remembered history of one's valued relationships to others, is being lost. The spreading of beta-amyloid plaque and tau tangles in the brain overwhelms cognitive memories. These memories are held in the hippocampus. Their emotional content is held in the amygdala, and there are synaptic connections to the prefrontal cortex, particularly the right hemisphere.

Neuroimaging (MRI technology) is used to identify major brain areas involved in the delusionary behavior common to neurodegenerative diseases such as Alzheimer's disease. Specific case studies in patients with delusions (including Capgras and Frégoli delusions) show right hemisphere lesions and hypometabolism in the right frontal and/or temporal lobes.[54] It has been found that an excessive release of the neurotransmitter dopamine is central to the neurobiology of delusions. Heightened output of dopamine leads to weakened activation of the PFC – the brain's reasoning center. Other studies reveal links between the damaged neocortex, both left and right sides, and hippocampal atrophy. Neuroimaging has also shown an increased thinning of grey matter in the cerebellum and parietal lobe before the onset of delusionary behavior.

Journal entries

The following journal entries show the presence of delusions as Alzheimer's disease advances in Edward's brain. The first entry shows an early sign of Frégoli syndrome. Paranoia sometimes accompanies delusion.

2019

11/18: My fourteen-day trip to Egypt begins. I booked the tour a year ago. I decide to let Edward drive me to the airport although he is supposed to stop driving. While I am boarding the plane, he gets lost driving home. We don't have GPS and he probably couldn't follow the navigation directions anyway. When I call him to see if he got home safely, he doesn't answer. I finally call our sons and tell them I don't know where their dad is. They call the police who begin to look for his car. I am tense with worry on the flight. Once I land in Egypt, I get word that he was found by the police several exits past our exit on the New York Thruway. John and his wife meet the policeman at the side of the highway and manage to get Edward home. James joins them; fortunately, both sons live within twenty to forty-five minutes from our house. Edward is unperturbed about the whole incident. He tells his sons that he stopped several times at gas stations and a pub to visit with old buddies from Pittsburgh. This is the first time that I encounter the delusions that occur in people living with Alzheimer's disease. It is early in the presentation of the disease. Incidents that represent a later stage can appear early on, like an Agatha Christie murder mystery where clues about the true nature of the murderer are teased into the early conversations and actions of the characters. Our sons and their wives tell me they will take turns staying with Edward while I am away. This gives me some relief.

2020

6/21: I have to take an item back to Lowe's. I retrieve Edward's Lowe's card from his wallet. He often sits on the bed and slowly goes through his bedside table drawer. He methodically removes wallet, photos, glasses' cases, small notebooks, extra shoelaces, and his phone (which he rarely uses anymore). Then he puts everything back in order. He yells, "Who's been riffling through my wallet! You have no right to go through my wallet! You have to ask permission!" I should have connected the dots here as there are few possessions that serve as reminders of his identity, particularly with his Lexus sold and gone. I tell him why I removed the Lowe's card and say he is out of line reacting to me as if I were a thief. But afterwards I understand why he reacted so vehemently. Delusions can show a person's hidden needs. His deluded belief that I was stealing his property shows his need to protect his identity, his sense of self.

8/31: We are watching TV news with our two cats. "Where's the other one?" he asks.

Astounded, I exclaim, "What other one? We just have two!"

He waves his hands as if to cancel his question.

2021

1/27: Words are coming out of his mouth that neither I nor he know where they originate.

After meditation he asks, "what about the burial?"

"What burial?" I ask.

"Forget it," he says, shaking his head.

Either he is momentarily delusional or there is damage to the speech areas which interferes with the production of thought into words – or both. As a caregiver, my job is not to react but to stay non-plussed, even inject humor, especially when his tone becomes truculent. I believe that something inside him knows he is acting abnormally, and he needs to justify it or cover it up.

2/26: Sitting by the fire this morning he fabricates a whole tale about entering a store where there was a line of wooden buddhas on a shelf. He said he asked the price of the last buddha. It was $5, and he bought it. We have an antique wooden buddha statue that sits on a side table. He bought it many years ago from a prestigious auction house in NYC. I tell him his story is a hallucination. He doesn't refute me. He just asks to hear the real story of how we got the buddha.

4/8: Today I see a stunning contrast between delusion

(from cognitive impairment) and cognitive lucidity. I wash some cloth finger puppets and put them on the wicker table outside to dry. Edward thinks they are cupcakes. Later he teaches me a prayer from Hindu Vedanta that he memorized years ago, and we reflect on it for ten minutes. Afterwards I say, "The prayer cuts through all that is transitory."

"Yes," he says, "that's because it is true. Yet there are corners of the self that do not receive it, until they do."

The prayer reads: *I am eternal, pure, liberated, formless, imperishable. My nature is one of infinite bliss. I am I, verily, the imperishable I.*

At dinner he asks, "when do we go back?"

"Back where?" I ask.

"New York," he says.

"We are in New York – this is our home," I say.

Things that are important to the person with Alzheimer's are retained, like the prayer he taught me. It could be that awareness of truth remains untouched by the mind-body's affliction.

5/9: After Mother's Day dinner at our house, I come down with a blocked small intestine. I am in the hospital for four days. Edward is staying with James and Ronnie. They tell me he is anxious, concerned about me, that he keeps asking the same questions. When I return home, James brings his dad back to our house. I ask Edward where he has been. He gives the name of a friend from the past. Though shocked at his answer I am getting better at not showing it. I give him clues about where he has been for four days until the memory of being at his son's house resurfaces.

2022

1/4: We park at the dermatologist's office in Monroe where we came a month ago for a checkup. He is looking at the lake across the street. He says, "last time we were here children were out in boats on the lake."

Surprised, I say, "no, those were geese and seagulls."

In bringing Edward back to reality, I see that he is not upset with the disparity between what he thinks he saw and what was really there. The possibility of fear being aroused when presented with an illusion did not occur in this instance.

1/25: Edward has lunch at James' house while I have a reiki appointment. When I ask him later about his visit, he says James' sons were there having lunch with them. I knew his sons were in school. Minutes later, he laughs and says that Jonah and Eli were not there.

***

Depression

The Columbia University Mailman School of Public Health reports that nearly one in ten Americans suffer from depression disorder. The United States, for all its wealth and quality of life, has one of the highest rates of citizens with depression. Mood disorders and bipolar disorder are linked to a greater risk of suicide. Being diagnosed with a terminal illness compounds the possibility that the afflicted person will become depressed. According to Kübler-Ross's research, in which she identifies five stages of the dying process in terminally ill patients, depression precedes the final stage of acceptance. The person living with Alzheimer's disease is depressed in a specific way, as death of the brain is a fearsome prognosis.

Kübler-Ross defines two types of depression: reactive and preparatory. Reactive depression happens when one loses someone or something of perceived value. For example, a woman who has undergone a mastectomy needs support from family and friends. Her self-esteem is shaken. She needs to be assured that she is still feminine. Preparatory depression is different. It is not based on recognition of past loss but of a future that contains many impending losses. With Alzheimer's disease, the person faces the destruction of his mind as well as the loss of those he loves and the life he lived. When people grieve about the emptiness they may feel as they approach death, as Edward did, and experience the feeling that they could have lived a fuller life, it isn't necessarily the time to cheer them up, says Kübler-Ross. Rather, the caregiver needs to quietly empathize with the sorrow that the loved one feels. By allowing the person to express that sorrow while sitting quietly with him, holding his hand, letting him know you are there until the end, the terminally ill person will find it easier to reach the final stage of acceptance.

When Edward would say, "I feel useless; my life is meaningless," I reminded him of all the good he did in his life. I said he can be thankful for several things: his service to the teaching through The School, his remarkable craftsmanship which he taught his sons and students, and the family who loves and appreciates him. Sometimes these inputs ameliorated the depressive mood. By reminiscing about our life together I encouraged us both to be grateful.

Gratitude is a positive emotion; it is called the natural anti-depressant. By focusing on what is good, what we have received that is good, depression and anxiety are reduced. Feelings of gratitude alter the brain's neural pathways by releasing the hormones dopamine and serotonin which lead to feelings of happiness. These feelings are ignited in the right anterior temporal cortex. The temporal lobe is involved in retaining visual and other sensory input in memory, along with their emotional evocations. Neuroscientists have discovered that grateful people have more gray tissue in the right interior temporal gyrus. Grateful people sleep better, are sick less often, are less affected by stress, and are generous and helpful to others because of their outer-directed nature. These behavioral traits generate a happy temperament.

Gratefulness arises naturally when one is mindful. In his book *Gratefulness, the Heart of Prayer,* Brother David Steindl-Rast starts by reminding his reader that gratitude comes spontaneously to those who are awake and aware. For example, when we are mindful, we can be continually surprised and delighted by the natural world. Seeing the first crocus of spring, or the golden light of morning streaming through the window after a night of heavy rains, are events that evoke a smile. Smiling is a gesture of gratitude. Thich Nhat Hanh was fond of saying that simple things, like smiling, boost the spirit and connect us to the world around us. Steindl-Rast reminds us that everything we encounter is a gift. Every given is a gift. Life is a gift. Remembering Steindl-Rast's philosophy, and guiding our attention to what is good, can extricate us from a depressive mood that seeks to claim our attention. Gratefulness is an essential practice for the person living with Alzheimer's disease as well as his or her caregiver.

In Edward's case, depression was often mixed with anger, frustration, and hopelessness. A few months before he died, Edward would often say he was depressed, had nothing to live for, and wanted to die. Both Eileen and Karen said similar things. Being aware, day by day, of the loss of one's mind with all its wondrous faculties of reasoning, contemplating, planning, and creating, must be excruciating. The emotional areas of the brain, like the amygdala, are still intact to feel these things, and the statement 'I want to die' shows an awareness of the progression of the disease. But awareness also validates the fact that the person is *not* the disease. The caregiver must continually remind herself and the loved one of this fact. Something conscious is watching the dying process unfold. In spiritual literature this something is called the Witness. It is the embodied Self. Michael often consoled his wife, Eileen, and himself, with the words, "You're still in there; you just can't get out." He told me he would lie down with his wife on the bed; they would hold hands as he told her the story of their lives together, and how love connected them.

Neuroimaging studies show that neurological disorders – ranging from depression to anxiety to schizophrenia – damage the prefrontal cortex. Lesions appear in the anterior portions of the frontal lobes. Lesions in the PFC can also result in apathy. Edward's repeated phrase, "I am useless," shows a lack of motivation which connects apathy to depression. In the later stages of the disease, when we went for abbreviated walks, he didn't look at the scenery. He looked down at his feet, concentrating on the strain of each step. Though I would say, "look at the tree, it's budding," he showed no interest. In his mind he was separated from his environment and could find no pleasure in nature. Stiffness and lack of balance in walking also indicated lesions in the motor cortex. The beta-amyloid plaque and tau tangles were spreading through his brain.

Journal entries

The following journal entries exemplify the well of depression in which the person living with Alzheimer's disease is apt to fall.

2020

10/3: Edward is sleeping longer, dozing off during the day. He seems to have lost interest in life. He no longer reads his School material and often picks up the newspaper only to put it down and doze off.

At lunch he says, "I'm depressed. I have nothing to do, nowhere to go, I can't drive."

I ask, "where would you go if you could drive?"

He doesn't have an answer.

2021

2/10: At lunch he says "I feel useless. I can't do anything, I can't drive. I feel like I don't belong anywhere, here, or anywhere. I have no home base." I try to console him saying we all feel isolated because of Covid. I try to interest him in renewing a routine of study, or taking up the Native American flute again, or brush painting which he used to enjoy. He says he wants to do these things, but then he doesn't do them. Is he aware at a deeper level that he cognitively can't do them? His normal drive and interest in outside things, in creative activities, are gone. He's trapped in a mentally limited environment without creative outlets.

6/15: After hours, even days, of mild behavior, he can suddenly become incensed over his limitations.

I call upstairs, "eggs are on!"

He yells, "F*ck!" He comes down in a foul mood, plops down on the chair and says, "this is criminal! I might as well be dead! I can't drive, I can't do anything. I know I'm in decline, but my brain still functions."

I restrain from mentioning Alzheimer's; it just makes him angry. "It would be good to have a hobby," I say.

"No, it makes me tired," he says. "I'm depressed, not bored. I feel trapped here. You can't do anything for me. I appreciate you taking care of the house." I wonder if I should ask the doctor for an anti-depressant. "I don't want your pity," he says, feeling my concern.

"It's love; I care about you," I say.

8/7: Mood swings change on a dime. He was tired, lay down to nap, saying, "I'm lost; I'm a lost man."

"You're not lost, you're here," I say. "I'm here with you."

"That's not what I mean," he says.

***

Towards the final year of Edward's life, agitation, anger, delusion, and depression coincide. The following journal entries introduce their confluence.

2022

2/1: An early lunch. It's Edward's birthday. I make his favorite cake. He talks about his son John as his brother, again.

I say, "you forgot to squeegee the shower door." (stupid of me).

He gets angry and starts to cry, saying, "I want to die!"

He waves me away. I come back ten minutes later. He is sitting down on the wing-back chair, sulking. I put my hands on his shoulders and say I love him.

He says, "it's been a difficult day for me." Then he looks at me, smiles, and quips, "and it's only eleven o'clock." At least he still has a sense of humor.

2/17: We are here in Florida for a month. I am thinking we should not have come. Edward's anxiety is palpable. The amygdala is on high alert. He's disoriented, confused about where he is. He gets alternately belligerent and depressed.

"I'm going home where I belong," he says. "I don't know what the f*ck I am doing here. I feel lost, displaced, hopeless, useless."

He goes to take a shower after supper. I remind him he showers in the morning. He explodes.

"It's your fault! Stop bossing me around."

2/18: We go shopping. "Whose car is this?" he says.

"Ours," I say.

"Where is Lyla?" he asks. This is the first time he doesn't recognize me.

"Who is she?" I ask, probing his memory.

"I thought she was my wife," he says.

"Yes, I am she," I say.

He looks stunned. "I feel like my head is screwed up for the last few months," he says.

"It's Alzheimer's," I say.

He doesn't react but says with some humor, "Ok, that's the same as having your head screwed up, brain scrambled."

A pause. "Are we married?"

2/20: While walking on the beach he says: "I need to call my brother."

"Who?" I ask.

"Ludge."

"He's dead," I say.

"Really? When?" he asks.

"Two years ago. We went to the funeral."

"I don't remember that," he says. "Does my family know I am here?"

What family is he talking about?

3/1: I have a 4:00 pm massage in Dunedin. I prepare wine and a snack for him in front of the TV. When I return, he is surly and uncommunicative. We eat dinner; he starts eating an avocado skin. I stop him, which annoys him. After we finish eating, I suggest that he can wash the dishes.

He shouts: "You do them! You've been out all day, just

thinking about yourself!"

I keep quiet. I know he feels rejected, inadequate. Now he can't discriminate between what's eatable and uneatable. Or is it his vision? Or both? This probably alarms him as I am certain he is aware that the disease is progressing.

3/21: On the way back to New York he is nervous, fearful. Each stopover is disorienting, though we've traveled this route many times.

"I live west of Pittsburgh," he says, hesitantly.

"No," I say, "we live together in Gardiner, New York. I'm your wife."

"You are?" he says, smiling coyly.

"Yes, fifty-three years," I say.

He attaches his identity to childhood places (Pittsburgh) and people (Mum, Ludge) that anchor him. People living with Alzheimer's are known to retain these long-term memories that have deep roots. They provide security – though I would say that fifty-three years of marriage should count for something!

"My family is almost gone," he says, referring to his Pittsburgh family.

"Our family," I repeat, "is you, me, our two sons, and their families."

"Where are they?" he asks.

"In New York, where we are going."

"Since when?" he asks.

3/22: As we travel, he obsessively checks his watch and opens the glove compartment where he put his wallet. His watch and wallet are like Linus blankets, to ensure his identity. Insecurity, anxiety, and fear put his brain on high alert. How do I help him get released from this obsessive-compulsive behavior?

3/24: Back home in NY, he is more relaxed. But at lunch two days later he says, "Aren't you glad to see me since you've been up here alone, and I've been in Florida?"

The next morning, he wakes up with a worried look. "I need to get a job," he says.

"Why?" I ask.

"We don't have any money."

I assure him we are fine financially. Money concerns begin to repeat themselves. This is part of his need for security. In cleaning up lunch dishes, he puts away his plate without washing it. It has syrup and grape stems on it.

4/20: I come home from grocery shopping; he says, "I'm not in good shape at all."

I ask, "What is it?"

"Deep depression, and you make it worse!"

I'm used to this technique of projection now; I don't react. At lunch the mood passes; he forgets about the altercation.

At bedtime he says, "I feel stagnant, useless; it's the most depressing time of my life."

For the caregiver, the downward spiral of delusion and depression in the loved one is a force that is difficult to confront, much less thwart. As a form of energy, however, it can be redirected into positive activities, using the faculty of imagination which all of us, including the person living with Alzheimer's disease, possess. The next chapter focuses on ways to elicit and grow this creative impulse. Creativity frees the soul to soar and experience pleasure, despite the limitations imposed by disease.

Chapter Five: **Nourishing the Soul**

One of Edward's favorite Shakespearean quotes was the speech to the players from *Hamlet*. He liked to recite it with full dramatic effect at gatherings of family and friends. It gave him pleasure, even into the later stages of Alzheimer's disease, to pull from memory the poetry of Keats and the dramatic soliloquies of Shakespeare. In part, the speech to the players reads:

Speak the speech, I pray you, as I pronounced it to you, trippingly on the tongue; but if you mouth it, as many of our players do, I had as lief the town-crier spoke my lines. Nor do not saw the air too much with your hand, thus; but use all gently, for in the very torrent, tempest, and (as I may say) whirlwind of your passion, you must acquire and beget a temperance that may give it smoothness.... Be not too tame neither, but let your own discretion be your tutor. Suit the action to the word, the word to the action, with this special observance, that you o'erstep not the modesty of nature....[55]

Just as we feed our bodies to keep them healthy, so the soul needs nourishment as well. Those living with Alzheimer's disease need an extra dose of soul food daily to keep the demons of anger, depression, anxiety, and morose feelings of defeat and isolation at bay. The caregiver also needs this food to strengthen her resolve to serve the person in her care and keep healthy herself. As the body of the person with Alzheimer's disease breaks down, and the brain is part of the body, the soul must be uplifted. Those things that are meaningful to the person, that stir the spirit, need to be discovered, drawn out and implemented by the caregiver. Even as the disease progresses – in fact *because* the disease progresses into more chaotic neurological territory – a balancing act that brings calm and joy to the person is necessary. Studies show that the brain, through its compensatory mechanisms – its neuroplasticity – will respond to this effort.

John Zeisel, sociologist and cofounder of Hearthstone Alzheimer Care facility, offers those living with Alzheimer's disease and their caregivers an innovative, compassionate approach to nourishing the soul. In his book *I'm Still Here,* Zeisel begins by assuring his reader that Alzheimer's disease is treatable, mainly through nonpharmacologic methods. The first thing to remember, says Zeisel, is that the person with Alzheimer's disease is still a person, even as the brain tissue deteriorates. This personhood must be remembered and respected. I would go further with the concept of identity. Deeper than personhood is the embodied Self or Witness, the I, which is beyond ego. As part of the mind, ego is an instrument that helps a soul get around in the world of matter, rather like a car for transport. The soul is that subtle, invisible, spiritual essence that passes on at death, leaving the mind-body behind. As Krishna explains to Arjuna, Spirit is "within all beings, too subtle to be perceived." [56] The imperishable lives within the perishable. What we are needs to be distinguished from what we have – a mind-body.

When the soul of the person living with Alzheimer's disease is nourished, body and mind are also nourished. A level of equanimity is possible. This refiguring of the body, mind, and spirit is achieved through the medium of the arts and spiritual practices. According to Zeisel, symptoms can be reduced and/or forestalled, especially in the early to middle stages of Alzheimer's disease. This is accomplished by discovering and drawing out inner strengths and aptitudes that produce joy, serenity, and a feeling of accomplishment in the afflicted person. Positive emotions are evoked as the amygdala assumes this affirmative role in emotional expression. It may be that an artist emerges, or a musician, or an actor. Through artistic endeavor – whether acquired during the lifetime or nascent – and through spiritual practices, the right hemisphere of the brain is stimulated. By means of the creative impulse, fostered in a calming environment by the caregiver, agitation is lessened even as the brain becomes more dysfunctional. As Siegel argues in his book *Mind*, the mind-brain naturally works towards integration, towards wholeness. Whatever strengthens the self-organizing ability of the mind-brain towards harmony is a positive energy to be cultivated, whether one is healthy or sick.

One of the physical gateways to access the creative impulse is the hippocampus. As memory's main storage facility in the temporal lobe, the hippocampus is affected early on in Alzheimer's disease by the build-up of beta-amyloid plaque and tau tangles. This build-up of toxic proteins causes short-term memory loss. However, there is evidence that valued memories are lasting ones. Valued memories can be accessed. In his experiments with stimulating the temporal lobes of epileptic patients, who were undergoing surgery and were conscious, Wilder Penfield demonstrated that the *whole* brain retains memory. Memory extends to a person's entire lifetime.

In his book *The Man Who Mistook His Wife For A Hat*, Oliver Sacks recalls Penfield's discovery and offers

162

examples from his own work with patients. One patient, an elderly woman, conversed with Sacks while experiencing an epileptic seizure. She spoke of vivid memories that took her back in time to her childhood in Ireland. She felt her mother's arms, heard her mother singing. Emotional, as well as cognitive, memories surfaced.

The discovery that memories are preserved in the whole brain points to the indestructible nature of awareness or consciousness. In the case of Michael's wife, Eileen, consciousness was demonstrated even during her last days. Bedridden and no longer speaking, apparently lost in a dream state, she was still aware through touch. She knew who was lying next to her. When her husband went to pull his hand away, she tugged at his thumb. On his last day, Edward heard my voice and knew it was mine; he felt my hands in his. These sensations of touch and sound are lodged deep in memory. They were our connection to survival and safety when we were babies, nursing at our mother's breast. We felt her body against ours, held her finger in our tiny hands, heard her croon lullabies to us. Even in the womb, when the cells of the fetus form a heart, it beats in synchrony with the mother's heart. We are in relationship even then.

The senses, writes Zeisel, are triggers for memory. This is not new to any of us. Every November, when I smell burning leaves piled in the neighbor's yard, I am immediately taken back to the house where I lived as a young girl. I feel the security of that time in my life. When we cultivate sensory awareness, we are in touch not only with the present but also the past. Time is a continuum of sensory awakenings preserved in memory.

Zeisel rejects the belief that those living with Alzheimer's disease become more and more like children. They do lose cognitive faculties, including a sense of time other than the present, much like infants. But they are adults, with long histories. They have many memories which serve as touchstones for exploring creative pursuits. These memories can elicit conversations. A person with Alzheimer's disease can be urged to share her story with the caregiver and family members. Edward's memories of his forty-four years of attendance at The School were firmly imprinted in his brain – and his heart. His delivery of the philosophy class four months before he died exemplifies this retained memory. Even as the neurodegenerative disease of Alzheimer's progressed, he could remember and converse about those memories in precise detail. They would evoke joy but also sadness because he knew he could no longer participate in that spiritually regenerative activity.

The development of latent talents and aptitudes in the person living with Alzheimer's disease delivers several benefits. Feedback from the caregiver, showing encouragement and admiration, is also important. The first benefit is a positive emotional reaction. As Hanson puts it, the person is *taking in the good*. The brain rewires, as the parasympathetic and sympathetic nervous systems come into equilibrium. As the creative activity is repeated and reinforced, neural networks in the cortex respond to the concentrated efforts of the blooming artist. A second benefit is the power of creative endeavor to give meaning and self-esteem to the person living with Alzheimer's disease. Even as he or she is experiencing the loss of cognitive capacities, an alternative way to experience the joy of life is burgeoning. Renowned mythologist Joseph Campbell was fond of saying, "follow your bliss."[57] He was advising his students to take up what most touches and awakens their hearts. It may be that the subtle heart is the soul.

We now examine how the arts and spiritual practices awaken, delight, and soothe those who are living with Alzheimer's disease. The bond between the afflicted person and caregiver is also enhanced.

The Arts

Another of Edward's favorite recitations was the poem by Keats which begins "A thing of beauty is a joy for ever: / Its loveliness increases; it will never / Pass into nothingness; but still will keep / A bower quiet for us, and a sleep / Full of sweet dreams, and health, and quiet breathing." [58] The arts are the contemplation of, and the release into manifest form, of beauty.

Physicist Amit Goswami describes the creative impulse as arising from nonlocal consciousness. Creativity is a mode of cognition that makes a quantum leap out of the limiting context of a person's conditioning in time and place. Goswami explains that creative work can fashion something new by means of insight. Creative work also has access to the collective consciousness of archetypal forms that encompasses the entire history of the human species. When the mind and heart are lifted out of the limited sphere of ego into unitary consciousness, creative germination takes place. Our higher self hears the promptings of the creative impulse and guides the work with ego as instrument.

Creative activity is stimulated mainly in the right hemisphere of the brain. Drawing, painting, the dramatic arts, singing, and playing an instrument are creative outlets that engage the *bottom-up conduit of perception*. They are based on sensory awareness. The creative impulse arises spontaneously, energizing the brain in ways that are fresh, nonlinear and nonlogical. To use a Zen term, creative activities arouse *beginner's mind.* There are no preset filters to determine the outcome of the activity. There is an absence of the usual dominance of the *top-down constructor* mode of perception which relies on learned experiences stored like files in the temporal lobes of the brain. As the person living with Alzheimer's disease loses cognitive faculties related to learned experience, the caregiver can elicit, from the person's history and tendencies, new avenues of creative expression. Such artistic endeavor enlivens the present moment which is the domain of persons with Alzheimer's disease. They feel the joy that accompanies the creative impulse. Edward's exuberant mood after his classes in Japanese brush painting expresses the power of the creative process to elicit positive emotions. According to psychologist Mihaly Csikszentmihalyi, pure enjoyment is a higher emotion than pleasure. Enjoyment, or satisfaction, arises when the mind-heart is fully attentive and absorbed in the creative process. There is then the possibility of a transcendent experience which Csikszentmihalyi calls *flow*.[59]

A story from the Hindu tradition describes the level of heightened consciousness that creates *flow*. There was a man gifted in the art of arrow-making. He would sit every day in his storefront studio in the village making arrows. One day, a wedding procession passed by. There was singing and dancing, as the people celebrated the bride and groom, with musicians playing their instruments. After the procession passed, a customer entered the arrow-maker's studio. As the arrow-maker turned his head to greet the customer, the latter said, "Wasn't that an exhilarating wedding procession?!"

The arrow-maker looked puzzled.

The customer frowned and said, with emphasis, "the wedding procession."

The arrow-maker shook his head. "I didn't hear any procession," he said. "I was attending to the point of this arrow."

There will come a time in the later stages of Alzheimer's disease when even the creative impulse is drained of its energy by the pull of sleep which overtakes the waking mind. But until that stage appears, bathing the soul in both the appreciation and practice of musical and artistic endeavors, theatre, and poetry can delight the mind and heart of the person living with Alzheimer's disease. Along with meditation and prayer – which will be addressed shortly – the arts enable the person to feel joy and personal meaning. The amygdala is calmed, allowing emotional energy to be expressed in positive ways. The brain is resting in the baseline responsive mode of the parasympathetic nervous system (PNS) – Hanson's *green zone*.

The arts also exercise the faculty of attention, as exemplified in the above story. The faculty of attention is housed mainly in the prefrontal cortex (PFC). Whatever the mind prefers and dwells on activates the relevant neurons and their networks in the PFC, translating them into action. The mind becomes still and attentive when it is usefully occupied. When the mind is trained to be still, under the direction of that which observes the mind – the higher self or Witness – it learns discipline and efficiency.

The Christian monk, St. Issac, said of this humble path of giving attention, "Love of wisdom means always to be watchfully attentive in small, even the smallest, actions.... Be sober and watch over your life; for sleep of the mind is akin to real death and is its image." [60]

Sacks recalls José, who lived in a clinic for the mentally ill. He was twenty-one, intellectually disabled, and diagnosed as autistic. He was considered by the hospital staff to be an idiot. José's parents vowed that, as a boy, José had been normal but over several years he had lost the ability to speak. He began to have seizures, sometimes twenty or more daily. His mental and emotional development atrophied. At age nine, José stopped elementary education. The doctor who was attending to him in the clinic thought that the electroencephalograms (EEGs) of his brain suggested the possibility of a temporal lobe disorder. This disorder impaired both his ability to speak and the development of conceptual and abstract thinking. He regressed into a noncommunicative, agitated state. When Sacks was called in to evaluate José, he discovered that the young man could 'speak' in a different, imaginative way. His mind operated beautifully in non-verbal, visual-spatial tasks like drawing. When he was a child, José loved the natural world and accompanied his father on walks where they would sketch scenes in nature. Sacks encouraged José to use this creative gateway to attain some measure of mental-emotional stability. José eagerly complied. Sacks watched the natural artist in José emerge and create, on paper, birds and trees with botanical accuracy and imagination. In time, José's agitation lessened. He even began to verbalize, hesitantly but determinedly. José was moved to a quiet ward, an environment that felt homelike and soothing. There was a garden outside his room where he could sketch what was there, like wildflowers, but also what he imagined in his mind, like a pond with fish. Though the damage to his temporal lobes could not be reversed, successive EEGs showed that the energy of his passion for drawing had replaced the violent energy produced by the seizures which lessened. The *bottom-up mode of perception* described by Siegel and translated by Sacks as *the power for the particular or the concrete*, had rescued José from a life of meaningless, terrifying isolation.[61] Drawing what he loved gave José a subjective reality which was just as real as the empirical, objective reality of a scientist.

José did not have Alzheimer's disease, but damage to the temporal lobes, which he did have, is one of the first neurological signs of Alzheimer's. As Zeisel recommends, it is vital to discover and elicit in people living with Alzheimer's disease latent talents, interests and aptitudes that can compensate for this damage. When Edward was diagnosed with Alzheimer's disease, we were in Florida at the Dunedin condo. I wanted to find a creative outlet for Edward. I remembered his delight in learning Chinese brush painting many years ago, so I suggested we check to see if the Dunedin Fine Art Center offered a similar course. The catalog showed an eight-week course in Japanese brush painting. Edward signed up and found that the teacher, an Asian woman, not only inspired her students to paint with abandon, but also encouraged them to meditate before practicing. This course turned out to be the highlight of the two winters we spent in Dunedin.

In her private practice, Reverend Diane favors a "soul enlightening" approach to healing the mind-body. Sensory communication is important. "For example, when you touch someone," she says, "they go into an altered state. Emotions come up so they can go deeper" to heal. She told me that working for Hospice helps her understand better the levels of consciousness. By listening to the terminally ill, she observes altered states. The patient and the caregiver "guide me," she says.

"I don't guide my patients. If I'm at all good at what I do I allow them to show me what they need. I'm looking for what gives them meaning, and I hold it up to the light. It may be family, work, art, social issues, politics, religion, spirituality. Whatever that is, I'm the student; they're the experts." [62]

In our conversations, Diane gave me several examples of her creative approach. One gentleman with Alzheimer's disease, whom she visited regularly, no longer spoke. She knew he loved music, so she tried greeting him by singing "hello, how are you, Mr. S.?" He then responded by singing back to her. Their conversation continued in song. Another patient, a woman with dementia from Parkinson's disease, was having trouble organizing sentences to convey what she wanted to say, so she spoke in metaphors. One day when Diane was visiting her, the woman broke out in a smile and said, "I like your aura." Diane took this to mean the woman felt comfortable, at home, with her. When Diane is with this patient, she remains present and attentive, waiting to decipher what the woman is trying to say but can't express properly. Diane believes that being fully present to a terminally ill patient is the portal towards forming a companionship that nourishes the person.

At our first meeting and interview, David described to me how his wife, Karen, became more withdrawn a year before she died from Alzheimer's disease. He had been feeling estranged from his wife for months. Karen's ability to outwardly connect with him, and with the world around her, was waning. He said he needed to find some way to communicate with her. A graphic artist by profession, David decided to share with Karen an artistic hobby. He made geometric designs on paper and gave them to her to color. This activity delighted her. "She would add a face or a banana; she'd add words from NPR radio or 'I love pancakes,'" he told me. "It was joyful and whimsical," he said, "and we could enjoy this activity together. She'd say, 'did I do that?'. 'Yes,' I said, 'we did it together.' She'd get possessive of it; it didn't bother me. I was so grateful for this time with her." [63] Below is one of their creations.

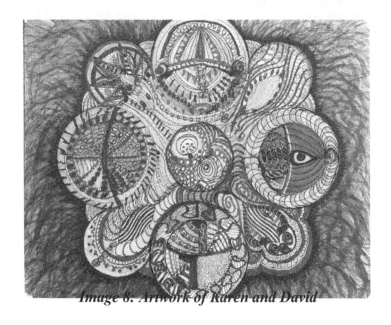
Image 8: Artwork of Karen and David

Both Michael and his wife, Eileen, were members of

The School for many years. We met there and became friends. Eileen had a beautiful alto voice. She and I were in the school choir together. One of her favorite songs was a Shaker song called 'More Love.' This suited her since she was a very loving person. Michael told me that the love she had for him and their adopted son, and the feeling of being loved, was total. It never left her. Michael recounted to me how, when she was diagnosed with Alzheimer's disease, she continued to play the piano and sing. There came a time, however, when she played the same piece over and over until even that composition faded from memory. Michael said, "I sang to her. I chanted Sanskrit sutras to her. She loved to hear the Yiddish songs that her father used to sing to her. I encouraged her to sing. Then her voice started to go, shreds and pieces. She would hold one note, one sound, for a long time." He continued, "She wore earbuds and listened to music. There were fifty songs I put together for her. She listened to music every day, up to the last two years."

Music is uniquely human. It is hard-wired into our brains along with language. Music is its own universal language, cross-culturally. Shakespeare wrote of the power of music to soothe the soul. In the *Merchant of Venice,* Lorenzo describes to Jessica how even wild horses are tamed, "their savage eyes turn'd to a modest gaze / By the sweet power of music: therefore the poet / Did feign that Orpheus drew trees, stones, and floods; / Since nought so stockish, hard, and full of rage, / But music for the time doth change his nature."[64]

Music can activate more parts of the brain than any other stimulus. It stimulates auditory, visual, emotional, and motor regions of the brain. These areas remain functional until late in the progression of Alzheimer's disease. In a three-year experiment with mainly Alzheimer's patients in a nursing home, social worker Dan Cohen introduced a personalized musical repertoire of songs to patients using iPods that he would place in their ears. These patients had withdrawn into noncommunicative isolation. Dan found this withdrawal to be a common phenomenon in the institutionalized atmosphere of nursing homes. Medical treatment is limited to sedatives and anti-psychotic drugs. To an onlooker, these patients appear vacant, lost, and dehumanized, but when they hear their favorite songs their posture and attitude drastically changes. They remember who they are. They come alive, their minds and hearts responsive to the music. Their faces glow, as recognition of the music, and associated memories of happy times which they treasured but had forgotten, awaken in their consciousness. They begin to sing and move their bodies to the music. They then willingly speak to Dan and the nursing home staff, relating with jubilation what they remember of the people and events associated with the music. They describe the feelings which the music evoked. One woman said the music made her feel whole again. A man recalled his Navy days. Crying tears of joy, he said the music made him feel good, like he had a date with a girl.

Dan's work became a documentary film called *Alive Inside*. Henry, an elderly black man, was the first person filmed. His bent head and blank expression turned into a joyful visage, pop-eyed and smiling, as he sang along with the Cab Calloway music he had always loved. He said that the music filled him with a feeling of love. His words rephrase Shakespeare who wrote in *Twelfth Night*, "If music be the food of love, play on." [65] As these men and women expressed their happiness in words and movements, their humanity reappeared. It had been veiled by the disease, the medications, and the cultural belief that dementia erases one's human standing. At the time the film was made in 2014, there was no financial support from the healthcare industry to make personalized music a therapeutic non-pharmacological treatment. When the film clip of Henry's 'awakening' went viral on social media, interest and donations skyrocketed. *Music & Memory* was formed: a non-profit organization born of Dan's mission to bring music therapy to the 26,000 nursing homes in America.[66]

Along with music are the theatre arts that can summon memory and provide a gateway to personal expression. Edward had a high EQ or emotional intelligence. His passion for the theatre and dramatic poetry were paramount interests that grew and deepened along with his commitment to the several roles he took on at The School: philosophy tutor, head of meditation, and head of physical work. He was one of a few men in The School who possessed a generous amount of *anima* or feminine energy. As psychiatrist Carl Jung points out, everyone has both *anima* (feminine) and *animus* (masculine) energies. Healthy individuation depends upon a person's discovery of the balance between these two energies which is inherent in his or her mental-emotional constitution.

Under the School leadership of Joy Dillingham, a gifted woman who combined intellectual acuity with artistic appreciation, Edward was given the opportunity to use his theatrical training to conduct acting classes. As a result of these classes, he directed two Shakespearean plays – *Hamlet* and *Romeo and Juliet* – assigning his students to various roles. The plays were put on at an off-off

Broadway theatre on the upper west side of Manhattan. Edward also organized and produced an arts and crafts festival at The School's retreat property in Wallkill, N.Y. for two consecutive summers. He was one of a small troupe of early risers who studied *tai chi chu'an* with Miss Dillingham on Wednesday mornings at 6:00 am. Edward also availed himself of classes in Chinese brush painting, offered by a Chinese American master. These rich experiences were imprinted in his memory. Even during the years of cognitive decline, if prompted, he would light up and describe these experiences. In the early stages of the disease, Edward and I practiced *tai chi chu'an* together. Because *tai chi* is a slow-moving, meditative exercise, he was able to follow and imitate my movements when he forgot the sequence of forms.

The Japanese brush painting class was, for Edward, an oasis of creative imagination that had been lacking due to his retirement from The School and his diagnosis of Alzheimer's disease.

On the next page is an example of his foray into Japanese brush painting.

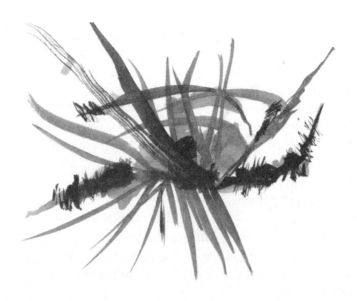

Image 9: Japanese brush painting by Edward

Journal entries

The following journal entries show Edward's delight in learning Japanese brush painting. Because it resembles Chinese brush painting, he was already acquainted with this art style. The first journal entry from 2019 shows how Edward was able to quickly discern the process of learning this type of painting. Of the two entries from the summer of 2020, the first shows a disconnect with the process and the second a refusal to continue painting. And yet, as the fourth entry shows, he still understands how to paint in the Japanese style but realizes that his ability to translate this understanding into action is no longer possible. The necessary neural connections between relevant regions of the brain have been interrupted by toxic proteins. The piano lessons, recorded in the journal entries, were less successful than the painting classes. It was a way, however, for Edward and me to be together using music as a cohesive tool. For us, piano lessons served a purpose like David and Karen's corroborative art project and Michael and Eileen's musical sharing.

2019

3/19: Edward begins taking a Japanese brush painting class at the Dunedin Art Center. He is avid in his daily practice. He likes the idea. He explains, with excitement in his voice: "Japanese brush painting is an emotional art; you get quiet and then let the brush paint whatever the heart wants to paint." I note that the paintings are abstract but can resemble features in the natural world, like trees, or even people. His artistic flair is on display, and the activity builds confidence. Perhaps the prominence in this form of art of allowing a spontaneous, emotional outpouring of creativity is easier and less stressful for people living with Alzheimer's. It avoids the strict discipline of logical and analytic left hemisphere skills. I bought the book *Drawing on the Right Side of the Brain* in hopes that he will read it.

2020

2/4: Edward is taking Japanese art classes again here in Florida. On the way home after his first class he says, "We drew a woman after she (the teacher) drew her on the board." After dinner I ask to see his drawings. He shows me two: a pitcher and a study of boxes utilizing the vanishing point.

I say in surprise, "I thought you drew a woman."

"No," he said, "we didn't."

Yet all the way home from class he was talking about it and when I said it must be hard to draw a person he said, "no, we just do the best we can to follow the teacher." Is this the beginning of delusionary behavior?

6/29: I suggest he continue with his brush painting here in NY. I suggest that we set up a work area in the garage. He refuses. I think he feels he has forgotten how to paint and is embarrassed to try. I begin to give him piano lessons. He's willing. From lesson to lesson he forgets almost all he learned in the previous session. He admits forgetting and is still not sure where middle C is, but during the lesson he has moments of clarity. Learning anything requires the ability to hold in memory certain knowledge and build on it. We have a lesson every other day. I encourage him, saying that learning piano is a good mind-body coordination exercise.

"Do you think I'll ever learn it?" he asks, with a child's innocence. "I forget all the time."

"It's worth it," I reply, "even as a present tense exercise. Maybe, with enough steady exposure, you can retain the basics."

8/28: He admires his twelve paintings that hang on the wall in the TV room in our Gardiner house. He asks me if I ever look at them.

"Yes, of course," I say. "They are hard to miss."

He laughs and describes with clarity how "brush painting is spontaneous, unplanned; a pattern arises. You don't do the action; it does itself." Edward understands this because an important teaching in The School is to stay present and attentive, letting the action take place without ego's interference.

Edward thinks he did these paintings here, in our garage, but I say, "no, you painted them in Florida where you took classes." His blank look tells me he doesn't remember attending those classes.

9/9: We are still doing piano lessons though each lesson disappears into the black hole of forgetting. We persevere.

10/3: At the piano he has spurts of matching the notes that are on the page to the keyboard, but he often reads what isn't there and goes down instead of up with the notes, or forgets which hand plays which staff. I realize that learning to play the piano relies on strong neural circuits between the PFC, visual, and motor cortices. An Alzheimer's brain can't handle this complexity.

***

Spiritual Practices

In September 2022, an article appeared in the Alzheimer's Association online library entitled "Measures of Religion and Spirituality in dementia: an integrative review." [67] The authors' intent was to evaluate whether people living with the terminal prognosis of Alzheimer's disease and other types of dementia benefit mentally and physically from spiritual belief and practice. The authors found that the need for meaning, particularly in a spiritual or religious way (the two were distinguished), was a common theme in the terminally ill. The authors also found that spiritual care for people with dementia was minimally present in the institutions where studies were conducted. This lack of spiritual care appeared to correlate with increased anxiety and depression in patients. The authors concluded that fostering a person's spiritual needs was associated with slower cognitive decline. They advised that more rigorous studies of people with dementia were needed to verify this conclusion.

Spiritual stimulation reinforces preexisting awareness which is the underlying essence of a person. Awareness is the vehicle by which his or her higher self is accessed. Spiritual care is especially important in a terminal prognosis. As Kübler-Ross discovered, acceptance of one's imminent death is the last stage of the dying process. It is a matter of common sense that a major task of the caregiver is to aid the person who faces the fact of human mortality by discovering his or her religious beliefs or the amorphous, but just as meaningful, spiritual inclinations.[68] The Hospice movement, initiated largely by Kübler-Ross, has brought both clinical and spiritual aid to the terminally ill, including those living with Alzheimer's disease.

In looking for what gives her patients spiritual comfort and meaning, Reverend Diane first acknowledges the "spark of the divine in each of us." [69] Because this spark expresses itself in each person differently, she believes it is her responsibility to bring that expression to light. Diane carries with her a booklet of prayers and songs from various religious traditions. She described to me a woman with terminal dementia who could no longer speak but wanted to pray the Hail Mary. The woman grunted the rhythm as Diane joined her with the words. Diane said that one way to facilitate a person's connection to the spark within him or her is through touch. When she touches the hand of the patient the soul of the patient meets and joins the caregiver's soul. "I am in awe of our physical being," she says. "It has a wisdom that is communicated through touch; it says, 'I feel your love.'" [70] This simple human companionship of being fully present to the 'other' as oneself fills the basic spiritual need to feel and know unitary consciousness.

Meditation

The treatment of body, mind-heart, and spirit is the objective of holistic healing modalities.[71] Beginning in the 1970s, Western medicine began to accept the legitimate health benefits of holistic healing methods from the East. These include reiki, Chinese acupuncture, Indian ayurvedic medicine, and meditation – both Hindu mantra meditation and Buddhist mindfulness meditation. The practice of meditation has been increasingly embraced in holistic medicine as an important component in the pursuit of physical, mental-emotional, and spiritual health.

In the 1970s, both Edward and I were initiated into mantra meditation at The School.[72] Daily meditation was a shared commitment in our fifty-four years of marriage. For Edward, meditation was the spiritual anchor which nourished him. The practice of meditation may have forestalled the arrival and progression of Alzheimer's disease. Not until late in the disease was his brain unable to concentrate on the mantra. As anyone who meditates knows, keeping the mind focused is not an effort reserved for people with dementia but is the challenge of all practitioners of meditation. Joy Dillingham used to remind her students that meditation is an elevated state of consciousness. We were still in the trenches, she said, *practicing* meditation. She was distinguishing a sustained, conscious attention on the object of meditation – be it mantra, sacred word, icon, breath, candle, or mandala – with the in and out experience of training the mind to be still and focused. The mind is easily distracted, so the purpose of practicing meditation is to train that which is aware, the Witness, to retrieve the wandering mind when it travels into a dream state.[73]

A story brings to life the struggle that a meditator faces when trying to keep the mind still. A man on horseback is galloping through a village. Another man who is standing on the side of the road shouts to the rider, "Where are you going in such a hurry?" The rider turns his head and, wide-eyed, shouts back, "I don't know; ask my horse!" Taming the mind is like taming a wild horse. The good news is that the mind can be trained to sustain its attentive capacity. It's not a matter of stopping movements in the mind. When we try that approach, those movements just multiply. Rather, it is a matter of being aware of what is going on in the mind yet continuing to turn our gaze back to the present moment. Gradually, mind and body learn to become still and present.

How often have we read a paragraph in a book only to realize that we don't remember what we just read? And so, we must read the paragraph again – this time with attention. In teaching classes of philosophy or in instructing students in how to work consciously, Edward was fond of asking, "where is the mind now? Where is your attention? How about now?... now?" When the faculty of attention is consciously joined to the body, specifically to the senses, then we are present. This is the practice of sensory awareness. In the present moment, we see and know we are seeing, touch and know we are touching, hear and know that we are hearing. The caregiver can help the person living with Alzheimer's disease zero in on this present moment, even as its existence is fleeting due to short-term memory loss. She can encourage him to be attentive to eating, bathing, walking, or any number of activities. She joins him in the practice of attention. Giving attention to everyday actions exercises the prefrontal cortex where the faculty of attention is located. Attentiveness can forestall toxic proteins from accelerating their attack on the neural circuits in this critical region of the brain.

Techniques of meditation – both religious and non-religious – vary. But all techniques have sensory awareness as their foundation, if they are authentic and potentially transformative. Meditation aims to lower stress by steering the amygdala away from its reactive mode, based in fear and aggression, to compassion for self and others. Meditation ultimately brings the mind to peace. This may take time, whether during a single practice or through cumulative practices that are regular in frequency and duration. Studies show that brain waves undergo transformation as the mind moves into quiescence. They transform from beta waves to alpha and theta waves. These waves are associated with inner peace and well-being. Blood pressure is lowered and, as breathing slows down, there is less oxygen consumption (this happens in sleep too). The mind-body rests in the serenity of the Self.

An important discovery for those living with Alzheimer's disease is the evidence through MRIs that meditation stimulates the hippocampus. Meditation enhances memory. It increases the capacity of the mind to learn and remember new things. Two studies confirm this benefit. In a 2009 study of forty-four long-term meditators, increased hippocampal and frontal volume of gray matter was observed. This increase in gray matter was particularly noticeable in the right hippocampus, right orbito-frontal cortex, right thalamus, and left inferior temporal gyrus. This finding revealed the ability of meditators to maintain emotional stability. They were able to stay emotionally stable by not reacting to stressful events, choosing positive emotional responses, and practicing mindful behavior.[74] A subsequent study in 2013 examined the MRIs of thirty long-term meditators and thirty controls, matched for sex and age. Similar results were observed. The left and right hippocampal volumes were larger in the meditators. Because meditation reduces stress, researchers concluded that increased hippocampal volume may combine a refinement of cognitive skills with better autonomic regulation and immune functioning.[75]

Many meditators use sound as a vehicle to keep the mind steady and focused. Sound has the power to heal. The word for power in Sanskrit is *shakti*. In Hindu mythological terms, Shakti is the wife or consort of Brahman, or God. She is the force of the forceful. Mantras are considered sacred sounds that have the power to guide the meditator towards Self-realization. Hindu Vedanta meditation uses mantras to that end. Centering prayer is a Christian method of meditation. It was developed by the Catholic monastics, Thomas Keating and Basil Pennington. In centering prayer, the spiritual seeker chooses a word that quiets the mind-heart. Choices can range from the name of Jesus or Mary to secular words such as *peace* or *love*. Buddhist meditation uses the imperceptible sound of the breath as a meditative anchor.

Sound penetrates the mind and registers in the brain

even as the neural connections atrophy in Alzheimer's disease. Edward's faithfulness to the morning and evening practice of mantra meditation nourished his brain with soul food. During the last year of his life, when his ability to focus on the mantra deteriorated into sleep, his mind still gravitated towards quietude. He loved to sit on the sofa for hours listening to the music of Mozart, Vivaldi, Gregorian chant, and Native American flute. I also gave him earphones so that he could listen to tapes of French philosopher Jean Klein, a teacher of Advaita Vedanta, whom he revered. The word *a-dvaita* means *not two*. Advaita Vedanta is the study and practice of the unity of the Self, the one consciousness that pervades everything. Edward had made these tapes by reading out loud from several of Klein's books, so he was listening to his own voice. If the caregiver can discover and make available to the person living with Alzheimer's disease the spiritual food he or she loves, then that person's soul is nourished.

Just as musical instruments need tuning, so the body – as a musical instrument – needs a tuning regimen of pure sound. Klein writes in his book *Living Truth*, "Every organ in our body is a vibration. All the organs in our body are like a symphony of sounds. When the organ loses its precise vibration, then it is ill..."[76] Healing through sound depends upon the establishment of tonal conjunction, or *entrainment*. The falling of the walls of Jericho, for example, may have coincided with a specific pitch and intensity of the trumpet blast. Clocks hung side by side will in time attune themselves to an identical swing of their pendulums. Deep in our collective unconscious are memories of tribal dancing around a fire to the rhythmic beat of the shamanic drum. The drumbeat has been likened to the human heartbeat. Using a microscope, one can watch as two muscle cells of the heart, each pulsing to its own individual rhythm, synchronize when they move closer together.

This urge to synchronize is the spiritual law of interconnectedness at work in the universe. It is interesting therefore that physicists have discovered a cosmic gravitational wave in the space-time background of the universe.[77] The ripples of the wave give off a humming sound that resembles the deep guttural sounding of Tibetan monks. The Big Bang, that launched the universe, was a sound. It is still vibrating. Hindu Vedanta describes this protean sound as OM. OM emanates from the *nada sound*, which is silent. The vital force in all beings, known as *prana* in Hindu Vedanta and *ch'i* in Chinese religions, is said to enliven all beings by its humming. All life forms are vibrating because of the collective humming sound of the universe. If we accept this unifying phenomenon then our worldview changes, from individual separation to collective community. Perhaps this humming sound is the source of the celestial music of the spheres.

Entrainment is central to new research in healing with sonic energy patterns. It has been found that the heightened state of consciousness which meditation promotes can be induced through technologies using sound. Sharry Edwards' groundbreaking *Bio-Acoustics* reveals that when a personal sound frequency pattern is disrupted by illness, health can be restored by exposing the person to his or her 'missing note' which has also been called the note of one's soul.[78] This information may seem esoteric and impractical, but it could be that when the caregiver sits in quiet contemplation next to the person living with Alzheimer's disease, their hands joined, they are experiencing a vibrational exchange based in love. They are immersed in healing energy.

Mitchell Gaynor, whose medical practice was transformed by his interest in sound therapy, says that the traumas and negative emotions that we carry in our bodies conflict with our true self, our essence, which is pure and tuneful. We become out of tune. He is convinced, however, that, through sound therapy, it is possible to consciously retune our bodies, hearts, and minds *at the cellular level* so that the divine musical score of our essence is restored.[79]

The brain has often been described in metaphoric terms as an orchestra. When healthy, its many diverse neural cells synchronize with each other to produce a healthy humming symphony that resembles the cohesive power and balance inherent in the music of Mozart or Vivaldi. If one section of the orchestra is off-key the harmony created by the whole orchestra is disturbed. The brain operates as an electrical circuitry of waves. Low-frequency theta waves coordinate the activities of disparate regions, bringing them into harmony and therefore optimizing brain functioning. In a recent study at Boston University, scientists discovered that they could improve working memory in elderly subjects by passing electrical stimulation through a skullcap to the brain. This stimulation amplified the theta waves through what is called rhythmic 'coupling' – a synchronization of electrical activity in frontal and temporal cortical areas.[80] Might persons who are at risk of contracting Alzheimer's disease benefit from such neural stimulation?

In another fascinating study, M.I.T neuroscientist Li-Huei Tsai found that when mice, whose brains were manipulated to show Alzheimer's symptoms, were exposed to a light and sound frequency of forty hertz, the rhythm of gamma waves in the brain was synchronized. Gamma waves are disrupted in people living with Alzheimer's disease. In the mice this gamma wave oscillation increased the activation of microglia cells which do the sanitation work of clearing toxins and regulating the immune system. Microglia cells were observed to effectively destroy beta-amyloid plaque and tau tangles in the brains of the mice. The gamma wave sounds also energized the brain's blood vessels, further clearing out these toxic proteins. Especially targeted were the temporal area, where memory is lodged, and the frontal area where decision-making and learning take place. The mice showed increased ability to learn and remember things. While mice are not people, it is tantalizing to consider how frequencies of sound and light might be used to reverse the progression of Alzheimer's disease.[81]

Mindfulness

Perhaps the most influential spiritual gift from the East to the West, in terms of the use of meditation as a healing modality in Western medicine, is mindfulness meditation. Mindfulness practice is the seventh step of the eight-fold path of Buddhism. The late Thich Nhat Hanh, Vietnamese Zen Buddhist monk and foremost teacher of mindfulness, introduced the practice into American culture beginning in the mid-1970s. It has since been popularized and is a household word. But what is mindfulness? Let us define it through examining an ordinary activity: driving. The mindful experience of driving is one of being outside the activity of driving – that is, *watching* the activity unfold – and simultaneously *participating* in the activity. While driving a car I am sensorily engaged in the action of driving: feeling the body seated in the driver's seat, feeling the hands on the steering wheel, foot touching the accelerator or brake with just the right amount of pressure, seeing the scene in front of the windshield and peripherally to either side. I am aware of whatever is happening outside of the car (other cars, road surface, traffic lights, et cetera) as well as what is happening inside, which includes the interior environment of my own mind, moment to moment. If I am daydreaming, I may cause myself and others harm. Thoughts will arise, like clouds moving across the sky, but if I am mindful, there will be an awareness of these thoughts and the ability to turn the attention away from their pesky intrusion and pay attention to operating the car. It will help if I meditate regularly because meditation practice feeds the practice of sensory awareness, or mindfulness, during the day. There's a good chance that the act of driving will be conscious rather than mechanical, mindful instead of mind-full.

One of the principal proponents of the application of mindfulness to medicine is Jon Kabat-Zinn, professor emeritus of medicine at the University of Massachusetts Medical School. In 1979, Kabat-Zinn founded the Mindfulness-Based Stress Reduction Clinic (MBSR) at UMass Medical Center. The aim of the clinic is to help patients cope with chronic pain using mindfulness techniques. Because there is a mind-body continuum, what we think affects how we feel, physically and emotionally. Kabat-Zinn uses a body scan to induce mindful relaxation of the body. He also teaches seated meditation, using the breath as a focus for the attention. Being mindful of the incoming and outgoing breath for short periods of time facilitates detachment and inner calm. For the patient, the physical pain may not disappear, but the relaxation of tension in the body, and the temporary arrest of negative thoughts about one's condition, help to decrease stress and make each day more livable, even enjoyable. The program continues to be a success.

In 2002, I attended a seven-day formation clinic in MBSR at the Omega Institute in Rhinebeck, New York. It was conducted by Jon Kabat-Zinn. He taught us how patients are trained in mindful meditation. They are instructed to watch the play of movements in the mind, the random thoughts and daydreams that spring up. This watching reveals the ordinary state of mind, of which we are usually not aware. Watching the mind induces detachment. It allows the patient to consciously let go of thoughts and sink into a state of relaxation. Watching the mind also fosters acceptance. The latter is important. As Kabat-Zinn teaches: "one accepts what is and loves it because it is." [82] Without acceptance, toxic stress levels rise in the body, exacerbating the illness. By accepting what is unfolding in the moment, the impulse to react from habit is replaced by creative response. Welcoming each moment, whatever it brings, with equanimity, is an art and a life raft to see us through all troubles.

Acceptance is a hard lesson to learn for the person living with Alzheimer's disease. If the caregiver can introduce a meditative practice that resonates with the person living with Alzheimer's disease, she is helping that person reduce stress and cultivate acceptance.

At about the same time that Kabat-Zinn was establishing MBSR, cardiologist Herbert Benson was investigating the calming effects of Transcendental Meditation, and other focused meditation techniques, at the Mind/Body Medical Institute at Harvard University Medical School. Benson discovered that the fight-or-flight response, so important to our ancestors, is overstimulated in modern society due to stressful factors. Hypertension was exceeding normal limits in his patients. He began advising his patients to meditate daily for ten minutes, morning and evening. He suggested that they begin with the breath as a focus and then follow that with a word that calms the mind. Benson called the exercise *the relaxation response* because relaxation of the mind-body is the inverse of its capacity to react to threat. In time, Benson broadened the meditative practice to include other mindful exercises like qi gong, tai chi chu'an, and yoga. As he monitored the physiological effects of meditation, he found a substantial decrease in the heart rate, breathing rate, and blood pressure in his patients. They were also experiencing emotional calm and a sense of peace that Benson associated with the altered states of consciousness that mystics of East and West have achieved throughout the ages.

Physiologically, meditation keeps the brain in the *green zone* – the place where the person living with Alzheimer's disease needs to reside. Chronic stress – also called *allostatic load* – puts the brain in the *red zone*, causing a flood of negative effects on the health of the body. Stress is the enemy of the person living with Alzheimer's disease, and a major challenge for the caregiver. Stress is a difficult condition to control even in healthy people, much less one who is aware that his or her brain is infected with toxic proteins. When the amygdala becomes revved up to react to threat the hippocampus and the PFC cannot do their job of inhibiting the amygdala's activation, because the neurons in these areas are atrophying. Moreover, psychological stress reduces the production of neurotrophins (brain derived neurotrophic factor or BDNF). BDNF, a key player in neural growth and resilience, protects neurons in the PFC. Stress also damages myelination. A person living with Alzheimer's disease shows myelin damage in the brain.

In contrast to these effects of prolonged stress, mindfulness training enhances the integrative neural links between the prefrontal cortex and other regions of the brain, such as the limbic system and brainstem. Mindfulness also strengthens myelination. When one steps back from events, so to speak, a space is created in the mind that allows physical changes in the brain to take place. The brain rewires itself through the mechanism of neuroplasticity. MRI imaging studies show that after a period of mindfulness training and application, the prefrontal cortex, including the anterior insular cortex, is strengthened in its task of regulating emotions, favoring positive emotions. The right side of the amygdala is stimulated and primed for empathy rather than fear or aggression. This strengthening of emotional health is important for the person living with Alzheimer's disease.

Empathy is the key emotional response in caring for a person living with Alzheimer's disease. Empathy is the ability to take on the perspective of the 'other' and thus feel what he or she feels. Only through empathy can the caregiver resist the urge to express her hurt feelings when the person she cares for projects his frustration or anger onto her. A valuable practice that strengthens the empathetic response is loving kindness meditation. Originally offered by Buddhist teacher, Sharon Salzberg, loving kindness meditation deepens this natural response of empathy which is based in the realization that there is no 'other.' There is only One. This feeling of oneness feeds and sustains the bond between the caregiver and the person to whom she gives care.[83]

Ecologist Carl Safina insists that all mammals share a spectrum of emotions, including empathy. Elephants, for example, will readily help each other. A researcher saw an elephant put food into the mouth of another elephant whose trunk was injured. In an experiment with rats, two tubes were presented to one of the rats. One tube contained chocolate chips and the other contained a caged rat. The free-roaming rat opened both tubes and shared the chocolate with his companion. Empathy makes us vulnerable in the sense that we open ourselves to the suffering of others. It is not easy to watch a loved one experience the loss of cognitive functions that we take for granted. But watch we must. Through being mindful we can respond with empathy, fueled by the knowledge that 'I am not this body, this brain, this pain of loss.'

It would appear counterintuitive to introduce mindfulness practice to someone who is very mindful of his terminal condition. Yet it is mindfulness that is the remedy. Paradoxically, mindfulness can make one feel both vulnerable and fearless. One is vulnerable because one wills that habitual opinions about oneself, one's spouse, and the world at large are put on hold, at least temporarily. One is receptive, porous as it were. But mindfulness also induces fearlessness. One wills to accept what is in the moment, including discomfort and pain, as a necessary prelude to change and transformation, even if that change is death of the body.

Research into mindfulness as an anti-aging tool has blossomed in recent years. In 1990, for example, only three journal articles referring to mindfulness studies appeared in scholarly journals. By 2018, there were 842 references.[84] Studies that explore the relationship between meditative practice and neuroscience are showing that mindful meditation can stem cognitive decline that comes with aging and its increasingly frequent bedfellow, dementia. In 2007, neuroscientist Dr. Clifford Saron and Dr. Alan Wallace, an expert on Tibetan Buddhism and founder of the Santa Barbara Institute for Consciousness Studies, led a study called the *Shamatha Project*. This study remains the gold standard of research into the benefits of mindful meditation. The study was conducted at a Shambhala retreat center in Colorado with sixty participants over a three-month period. It consisted of in-depth instruction and practice of a variety of intense meditation practices, including loving kindness meditation. In a comprehensive scientific measuring of the results, significant findings emerged. These findings included the following: improved attention (with less mind wandering and improved response inhibition), a lessening of anxiety, depression and other negative psychological states, a feeling of well-being, sympathy when shown disturbing film clips of people in pain, and evidence of an increase in telomerase activity. Telomerase is an enzyme that lengthens telomeres. Telomeres are bits of DNA that form protective caps on chromosomes in our genes. Scientists compare them to the plastic coverings on shoelace ends that prevent the laces from unraveling. Longer telomeres slow down the aging process. They prevent harmful chronic inflammation and a weakened immune system that can afflict the elderly. The meditating participants had longer telomeres in their immune system cells than the control group where no change in length was noted. Apparently, as we get older, telomeres tend to shorten, contributing to age-related illnesses like osteoporosis, cardiovascular disease, dementia, and diabetes.

In their 2017 book *Altered Traits*, neuroscientist Richard Davidson and psychologist Daniel Goleman present findings from their investigation of what Davidson calls *contemplative neuroscience*. They found that what begins as a neurologically altered state in the brain, resulting from meditation practice, can become an altered trait. A permanent rewiring of brain circuitry can take place. Because neuroplasticity is a property of the brain, the structure and waves of the brain alter when imprinted repeatedly with meditative exercises. The effect is enhanced physical and psychological health. The capacity to sustain a lifestyle of detachment, equanimity, and empathy grows. The authors mention several brain areas that are calmed and brought to equilibrium, fostering a quiet enjoyment of life. The amygdala is one such area; another is the nucleus accumbens which plays a role in our attachments and addictions. Long-time meditators have less gray matter in this region.

In their examination of the MRI brain scans of long-term meditators, Davidson and Goleman found that certain parts of the cortex were thickened. Specifically, the anterior insula and areas of the prefrontal cortex, which sense the body's interior state, were thickened. This thickening of tissue was related to a slowing down of the breath (less oxygen intake) and a relaxation of tensions in the body. Evidence of increased folding of tissue in the top of the neocortex was also observed. The researchers wondered, is a younger brain being created? Is an altered trait being established by sustained practice? When a group of yogis were similarly tested, evidence of gamma waves appeared. Gamma oscillations are connected to enhanced neural connectivity, leading to elevated cognitive and emotional functioning.[85] Yogis are defined as practitioners of yoga meditation who have attained sustained levels of heightened consciousness. The waves produced in the brains of the yogis were not limited to periods of meditation but were also observed in their everyday activities. Davidson and Goleman report that they saw and felt the ease and effortlessness that emanated from the yogis. Their lifestyle of equanimity was palpable.

One of the teachings of The School is that regular meditation practice for a half hour, twice a day – morning and evening – will in time spill into the other twenty-three hours of the day, strengthening one's ability to sustain attention and remain present and relaxed. This sustained attention is mindfulness. Mindfulness is a form of health because it connects us – body, mind, and spirit – to our source. The class that Edward taught four months before he died was a snapshot of forty-four years of practicing mindfulness. He was in an altered state of effortless awareness in which his mind-brain gathered the gems of his understanding of the teaching and offered them in dialogue to his audience. We, his students, were drawn into this sphere of sustained attention, induced into the same state of calm and certitude from which he was speaking. Our minds were in synchrony. If there was a genetic component in Edward's contraction of Alzheimer's disease, it may be that the forty-four years of meditative practice kept the disease at bay for a long time. As research into the relationship of meditation, aging, and dementia continues, it is heartening to hope that meditation may be found to defer, and even prevent, the development of Alzheimer's disease, especially if signs of the disease are diagnosed early.

Inclusion of the arts and spiritual practices in the

treatment of Alzheimer's disease not only nourishes the person living with the disease but also strengthens the relationship between the afflicted person and the caregiver. The bond between them deepens, particularly if the caregiver engages in these activities with the loved one. The arrival of Alzheimer's disease in a relationship introduces a new and formidable element that will change and test the relationship. Adaptation is required, and this falls to the caregiver to achieve. Alertness and flexibility will enable him or her to learn the deft and fluid dance choreographed by Alzheimer's disease. In the next chapter, we will examine how the special relationship between the caregiver and the person living with Alzheimer's disease develops and changes.

Chapter Six: **Changing Relationships**

Traveling through the minefield of Alzheimer's disease is as much about the caregiver as the person with Alzheimer's. Although this chapter will be examining the changing relationship that will occur between spouses, the main themes will apply to other dual roles as well, such as child/parent and nurse's aide/patient. A severe health crisis – indeed, any crisis – challenges a close relationship. It sets up stress for both people who are entering an unknown landscape mentally, emotionally, and spiritually. A marital relationship of many years is set in its ways like the people who created it. The dynamic of this old relationship remains, with its scars and its beauty, but now it is shaken loose and overlaid with new and sometimes abrupt changes. Personality flaws are exposed. Guilt and regret can arise from memories of these flaws colliding in past actions. But the crisis also presents opportunities for both people to see and overcome old impediments that have impaired personal growth and even stunted the relationship in certain respects. New adaptations may be required. Because the person living with Alzheimer's disease is increasingly unable to modify his behavior, it falls upon the caregiver to make the necessary adjustments to keep the relationship stable.

Spiritual growth can be stimulated if each partner is willing to admit his or her own flaws, while resisting the urge to criticize the other. Criticism is a form of projection. It may be that two people come together and form a long-term relationship to untie each other's karmic knots. The temptation to use marital conflicts of the past as ammunition in the present prolongs those conflicts and solidifies them. The past is in the present. If we pluck its bitter fruit and use that negativity against one another, then we miss the opportunity to use the present to change the relationship for the better. Memory is spotty and incomplete. It cannot capture who we were over the long string of married years, nor why we chose certain actions. A health crisis can either sink both spouses into recrimination and negativity or liberate them from the bondage of the past to chart a new path forward.

To help relieve symptoms of Alzheimer's disease in the loved one, and minimize occasions that might produce stress, it is important for the caregiver to stay in underlying awareness, or mindfulness, as much as possible. Staying mindful will also relieve the stress experienced by the caregiver who is called upon to be patient and calm, often over a period of years. Cultivating patience is not easy because we desire that the person be as he or she used to be. For example, the loved one will ask the same question over and over. The caregiver learns not to say, "I just answered you." Rather, she gives the answer again. As Jesus said to Peter who asks him, "Lord, how oft shall my brother sin against me and I forgive him? Until seven times?" Jesus replies, "I say not unto thee, Until seven times: but, Until seventy times seven." [86]

The caregiver will make mistakes. Caring for someone with Alzheimer's disease is not a school for the formation of saints. However, there is a learning curve that can deliver positive results. Again, patience and calm acceptance are the virtues to be practiced in service to the beloved. As Hamlet said to his mother, Gertrude, "assume a virtue if you have it not." [87] These virtues will blossom because they are innate. Beneath them is the awareness of the Self, within both partners. Awareness is the subtle substance which connects the person living with Alzheimer's disease to the caregiver, through the medium of love. Resting in awareness generates the healing energy and sustenance that both the caregiver, as lover, and the cared-for, as beloved, need in their joint journey.

True service is selfless. It bypasses ego's intentions and desires. It is free and pure. Service is the ultimate human function. Rabbi Abraham Joshua Heschel teaches that we are saved from the sins of arrogance and small-mindedness when we realize, with gratefulness, that service to the Creation is the gateway to the perfecting of the soul. He writes:

Amidst the meditation of mountains, the humility of flowers – wiser than all alphabets – clouds that die constantly for the sake of His glory, we are hating, hunting, hurting. Suddenly we feel ashamed of our clashes and complaints in the face of the tacit glory of nature. It is so embarrassing to live! How strange we are in the world, and how presumptuous our doings! Only one response can maintain us: gratefulness for witnessing the wonder, for the gift of our unearned right to serve, to adore, and to fulfill. It is gratefulness which makes the soul great.[88]

Serving the needs of the 'other' as myself in a different body is a form of sacrifice, of making sacred one's actions, without thought of reward. At the clinic she founded in Calcutta, India, Mother Teresa taught her Missionaries of Charity that serving the poor, the sick, and the dying with a fulsome heart was the same as serving Jesus. In the *Bhagavad Gita*, Krishna speaks of sacrifice. He says to Arjuna:

Whatever thou doest, whatever thou dost eat, whatever thou dost sacrifice and give, whatever austerities thou practisest, do all as an offering to me. / So shall thy action be attended by no result, either good or bad, but through the spirit of renunciation thou shalt come to Me and be free.[89]

Ordinarily, a healthy spousal relationship has its outbursts followed by its mending rituals. The curves of the relationship become familiar, expected even. But when one spouse is ill, especially if the illness is terminal, old wounds and sensitivities are magnified. In the person living with Alzheimer's disease, the amygdala, the seat of emotional response, remains intact deep into the progression of the disease. This part of the brain becomes increasingly unregulated and subject to volatility due to the weakening of the inhibitory functioning of the hippocampus and the PFC. In response to these neurological changes which the person living with Alzheimer's disease cannot control, the caregiver must develop new skills, like a lizard growing a new tail. Patience, kindness, even sometimes the silence of non-reactivity – not the silence of criticism – needs to be cultivated for the relationship not to descend into chaos. The vow to be true to one another 'in sickness and in health' is tested. When I was able at times to tell Edward for the twentieth time where a glass belonged in the kitchen cabinet, with complete neutrality of tone, without a trace of hidden impatience or criticism, I knew this achievement was an act of love. His illness allowed me to see my biggest faults: a tendency to bossiness and a compulsion to control events. The danger of falling into this pattern was exacerbated by Edward's slow pace of comprehension. When negative emotions were veiled with forced 'niceness' on my part, Edward's own capacity to be sensitive to my inner world would emerge to deliver a sharp rebuke. Spouses, as well as parents and children, carry inside them a silent, shared energy that is constantly being communicated between them, whether intended or not.

Because the amygdala is still functional, even as neural connections between regions of the brain fray, the person living with Alzheimer's disease is still acutely aware of his own emotions and those of the caregiver. His emotional sensitivity must be matched by compassion in the spouse. In the Hindu and Buddhist traditions, the practice of compassion is called *ahimsa*. The word translates as compassion and non-violence. When the afflicted spouse suddenly projects anger at you, his caregiver, the tendency to defend yourself is strong. You come to understand that his anger is born of fear and frustration. Responding rather than reacting is key to de-escalation of the emotional outburst. If I am present, I may be able to find that space of quiet in the mind to digest why he is reacting angrily and respond with love. Love can never be destroyed by dementia. When we say 'I love you' to each other, all the prickly sensations of resentment, hurt, anger, and sadness melt away. David recounted a time, after Karen received the diagnosis of Alzheimer's disease, when her reaction abruptly changed from acknowledgment to fear and denial. When he suggested that they could hire help she resisted strongly, lashing out at him. He had suddenly become an adversary rather than her advocate. But outbursts like this, he said, could be followed quickly by "'I love you; thank you.' When she insulted me, I first tried to counter her falsehoods, but then I realized I couldn't reason with her." [90]

Michael told me that his relationship with Eileen became strained because of the length of her illness – ten years. He had to be constantly ready for abrupt changes in behavior that would overcome her gentle poise and loving nature. Michael admitted that he was not always able to restrain his own anger and disappointment as he watched his wife become a shadow of herself. He described to me the changing relationship, and the difficulties he encountered:

While it was going on, how I felt and what I did was not always in tune. I saw a therapist who helped. And I talked to a friend, a psychologist, a lot. I went through a lot of misery, a lot of loneliness, like eating at the table with her without conversation. Driving alone, I would sometimes scream. I got past 'why is this happening to me?'. I meditated regularly, attended class, and tutored a course on happiness no less! In the deepest part of me there was contentment, and I felt protected after she died. I experienced loss and grief, but this had started years before; it was parceled out already. Our relationship felt like a painting, with flakes falling off. You go through a spectrum of emotions – rage, anger around the grief. But I never blamed God. When I was with her there was love and sadness.[91]

Michael told me that even as Eileen sank into periods of despondency, rage, and withdrawal, she never felt unloved and never stopped loving. Even towards the end of her life, he knew she was "still in there and still loving."

Whenever Edward vented frustration and anger over his decreasing independence, I knew I had to rise above the friction that tore at our relationship. When he could no longer drive or pay the bills or do simple carpentry tasks, he felt diminished. His manhood was threatened. I was Edward's sounding board and sometimes the object of his projection. He would get defensive to protect himself, while I struggled to be patient and compassionate. One way to shift the marital dynamic was to let him do as much as he could in simple activities without my interference. At meals, I needed to get used to Edward sometimes eating with his fingers. When his clothes were laid out for him in the morning, I let him put them on. When buttoning his shirt, I waited to see if he could do it, and only if he became frustrated did I step in, kindly. One morning, as he began to put on his tank-style undershirt, he chose to put his head through one of the armholes. I helped him wriggle out of the tight fit and made light of the error. We laughed about it.

Like Michael and David, I was also dealing with loneliness. The man with whom I used to have stimulating conversations about politics and spiritual teachings was not forthcoming. Edward was silent, not because he didn't want to converse, but because he couldn't. The physical effects of Alzheimer's disease also lower the sex drive. A withdrawal of sexual relations strains the spousal relationship. The bonding intimacy of touch is a human need that satisfies not only one's libido but the mental-emotional reservoir of love that generated the relationship in the first place. The withering of intimate relations must be particularly distressing for spouses who are dealing with early-onset Alzheimer's disease, which affects approximately 5-6 per cent of Americans, ages thirty to sixty-four.

As a spouse, I learned new housekeeping tricks. When we moved to a one-story ranch, Edward was entering the latter stage of Alzheimer's disease. I needed to create an orderly, calm environment. I removed certain pieces of furniture, like an ottoman and coffee table, because he might bump into them and fall. We walked around the interior of the house every day to familiarize him with the layout, which he would forget. The stone patio in the back of the house is broad, rising about a foot off the ground. It provides a quiet place to sit and look out at the vast backyard of old maple trees, dogwood, viburnum, and boxwood. But there were no railings bordering the patio. To prevent a fall, we had railings installed.

As caregiver, I had to take on new roles besides *spouse*. These roles required a cram course in psychology, biology, and spiritual counseling. I became *parent, nurse, spiritual advisor*, and *muse*. The role of parent is a difficult one because the husband is not your child, and you are not a parent to him but his wife. Yet, just as a parent is her child's first teacher, teaching the child how to do simple things, so to the same extent I had to help my husband relearn how to dress, how to navigate the layout of the house, how to bathe, brush his teeth, and wash his hands after using the toilet or before a meal. The dynamic of wife playing the role of parent also at times triggered the layered emotional ties that Edward had to his mother, evoking both positive and negative feelings. David recounted how his relationship to Karen gradually changed to one of parent-child. He was grateful for the artwork, in which they collaborated, for it resuscitated the husband-wife, artist-to-artist relationship which had been hidden and degraded by the disease.

As nurse, I had to oversee medications and in the later stages help Edward eat, bathe, dress, and go to the toilet.

As spiritual advisor, I had to remind Edward of our true identity as spiritual beings. Sometimes he reminded me. As muse it was important that I counter his tendency to sink into depression by encouraging him to tap into his creativity. The creative impulse manifested periodically in Japanese brush painting and his attempt at learning to play the piano. When our sons and their families came to visit, I encouraged them to engage Edward in conversations that reawakened colorful memories of his past achievements in theatre and how his love for the Teaching inspired many students in The School.

In all these roles that a caregiver must play, it is important to be honest – that is, to be yourself. Again, the person you are caring for has feelings, and through feeling, knows if what you are saying is truthful and honest. There is some debate about the nuances which arise in speaking the truth. As the journal entries have shown in previous chapters, Edward did not want me to say that he had Alzheimer's disease. I learned to be silent when he complained of the changes he was observing in himself. There came a time, however, when he could accept the truth about his condition. I also discovered that speaking the truth in a way that is accepted means not necessarily what you say, but how you say it. How we speak the truth, so that it penetrates the listener's heart, depends on our own practice of mindfulness and compassion. It is mindfulness that attunes the caregiver to her own sensitivity to the needs of the person she is caring for. It is through this sensitivity that she measures out the truth to fit the occasion. Reverend Diane spoke of a woman in the later stages of Alzheimer's disease who had lost her husband several years before. One day she asked Diane where her husband was because she missed him. Diane had to decide whether to say he had died or to say he was at the store shopping. She was ambivalent about how to respond. She chose to say the husband was at the store because she could see that the woman was anxious and fearful. She also knew that the woman would promptly forget the exchange between them.

Incidents arise that challenge whether one speaks truthfully or dodges the truth. In his book, *I'm Still Here*, Zeisel argues that little lies, or *fiblets*, are permissible if they fulfil certain functions. They should accord with the reality that the person with Alzheimer's disease has adopted, prevent the eruption of painful memories still held in the damaged hippocampus, and reduce anxiety. Zeisel gives the example of a person with Alzheimer's disease who feels abandoned, even though she is receiving compassionate care. Rather than say, 'no, you are not abandoned; look at the care you are receiving,' a better alternative is to empathize with her feeling of being abandoned because for her it is real.

A trickier problem is how to deal with the delusions of a person living with Alzheimer's disease. On a summer evening in 2021, Edward was meditating inside while I was sitting on the patio meditating. After meditation he asked me if the others who were meditating with me left. I said no one was out there with me. My honest response satisfied him. This was the first time he mentioned imaginary people. In their book *Living with Alzheimer's and Other Dementias,* Amy Newmark and Angela Timashenka Geiger present a compilation of short essays by caregivers. One of the subjects that these essays address is the caregiver's response to delusionary behavior.

In one essay, a woman with Alzheimer's disease who

resides in a nursing home is wheeled into the dining room by a new nurse. The woman suddenly stops the wheelchair, clutches a doll in her arms, and refuses to go into the dining room. A more experienced nurse walks over to the woman and says that the baby she holds is hungry. She suggests they go together into the dining room to get the baby some food. The woman smiles and relents. The nurse's response shows that there are creative ways to deflect and redirect the afflicted person's fears and anxieties by entering her imaginary world.

In another essay, a son speaks of visiting his father who has Alzheimer's disease. The father is still living in the family home. When the son arrives, the father tells his son to take him home. The son, realizing that his father has entered a more advanced stage of the disease, tries several strategies to convince his father that he is already at home. This effort includes showing his father the family photos on the mantle. But his father says he doesn't know those people. The son finally comes up with a creative solution. He takes his father outside, they get in the son's car, and he drives his father around the block and back to his house, which his father now recognizes.

In a third essay, a mother living with Alzheimer's disease becomes childlike and forgetful. The daughter writes that she and her mother enter the living room. The mother hallucinates, seeing babies sitting on the sofa. Her daughter uses humor to deal with her mother's fantasy. She asks her mother to point out where the babies are so that she won't sit on them. They both break out in a healthy bout of laughter. At a deeper level it appears that the mother knew that what she imagined wasn't real.

A final example from the book offers the perspective

that a person engrossed in delusions should be humored, even rewarded, and her imaginary world affirmed. In this essay, a mother with Alzheimer's disease insists that she was a fighter pilot who rescued children during a war. The daughter, who writes the essay, describes how she decided to celebrate her mother's birthday by inviting relatives and friends to a party for her mother. During the celebration the daughter, amidst a clapping audience, presents her mother with a medal of honor, made by her granddaughter. This recognition of the mother's imaginary heroism makes the woman happy. But one could argue that this ruse goes too far. To lie in this way is to degrade the humanity of the person living with Alzheimer's disease. An equally creative but more truthful response to the mother's need to be recognized could have been devised. The daughter could have still given her mother a birthday party. At the party, each attendee would present a card expressing, through personal example, praise for one of the mother's good qualities. The cards would be read aloud punctuated by applause after each one is read.

Journal entries

The following journal entries from 2019 to 2022 are selected to show the twists and turns of the changing relationship which Edward and I experienced. Sometimes there were surprises, stimulating a new set of responses.

2019

7/10: When I 'correct' Edward for putting the garbage bags in the recycling container he hears a subtle tone of criticism in my voice. He carries this insult to the front porch where we sit down to talk.

"You don't respect me," he says. "I've given you this

house, everything. Maybe I should leave." He gets defensive, sits glum and brooding, and can't get out of the funk. In these times, I can only be silent. Finally, he says, "I'm not happy."

My heart drops. "I know," I say. "There are things you can do, your brush painting for instance. When you feel this anger, you blame me. It's projection."

He is silent.

"You have everything anyone your age would give their eye teeth for, even with Alzheimer's," I say.

"Don't say that word!" He glares at me. A few moments pass. I wait. Finally, he pulls me onto his knee, but no apology for his anger.

8/3: Edward rinses glasses instead of washing them with soap. I gently remind him. He gets angry, then later reaches out, apologizes, and we embrace.

8/9: I talk to Edward about properly repairing the chair leg of the sofa. He insists that the makeshift fix is fine – very unlike him. "I've worked all my life, I don't want to now," he says. I think he is hiding the fact that he knows he can't do this work anymore. It is a matter of pride. I must honor this vulnerability and help preserve his self-worth.

8/20: I fell and fractured my ankle. Edward has to do housework and cooking. He forgets which buttons to push to do the laundry. Several clashes occur when I 'correct' him.

He says, "you're accusing me. I hear it in your voice."

Was accusation in my voice? I don't know.

While he is pouring his tea I say, to be helpful, "your juice is over here."

"Can't you see I'm pouring my tea," he retorts testily. "It's you, you are doing this to me," he says, glaring and pointing his finger at me.

Later we talk and mend the rift. He says, "we can't do this to each other." I am surprised at this admission because I am usually the one to reach out.

9/23: He feels imprisoned in his own house because he can't drive. He is feeling more and more defensive and sensitive. I have to be careful. Even if criticism is not the motive, he can imagine it and react with anger, even paranoia. Our fifty-three year marriage comes under attack with judgments about the past. Past conflicts rise to meet perceived insult or criticism in the present.

This morning, I call upstairs, "It's cold down here; can you come down and make a fire?"

"Is that my duty?" he retorts. I know this reaction comes from a longtime feeling on his part of being ordered around, sometimes warranted, though not in this instance. When he comes downstairs, he hugs me and goes to make the fire.

Today he wants to talk about these small incidents that accumulate. I explain that the sudden mood swings and feeling slighted are exaggerated and even sometimes imagined, because of Alzheimer's. He doesn't like to talk about that.

"I don't feel sick or different," he says.

"It's mental-emotional," I say.

"We must stay aware and be loving," he says. I nod in agreement.

I feel close to him after these words. Even with forty plus years of practicing the teaching of staying present and observing one's actions, it is hard now, for both of us. Reactions may not yield to awareness. A tendency to go with a negative pattern is ascendant.

2020

1/4: Edward doesn't like the pill dispenser. He says he has his own system. When I point out the usefulness of the dispenser, he gets angry and says, "we never talked about this…" (we did) "…you're taking over!" It's true; I am taking over. He is becoming more dependent on me, and he hates it. It's like I'm his mother, but he's a grown man. How can I assuage his frustration? Holding his hand, hugging helps – if he lets me.

4/17: We get into an argument when he drops a saucer and it chips. He gets upset with himself and me. We sit down to talk. He says I make him nervous, always watching him, criticizing, and judging him. I say he is wrong, that this is defensiveness against the disease itself. "This is Alzheimer's speaking," I say. "I am not making you nervous, you are reacting to what the disease does. It uses our personal flaws to create a wedge between us. Blaming me comes out when you feel exposed and weak. Fight this; it isn't you." He listens. The rest of the day he is calmer, more helpful around the house.

5/12: I am getting his morning tea ready. I call upstairs to see if he is out of the shower so I can time the tea. He 'attacks', saying, "you are always herding me!". When he

212

comes down to the kitchen he has forgotten the exchange. I am doing a lot for him, and I feel unappreciated. Then he says, "thanks for the tea." He is conflicted, realizing his dependence on me but hating it at the same time. I have to back off, not take his comments personally when he gets touchy and paranoid. This time he takes the tea and says, insightfully, "It's all reactions; me to you, you to me." He's right.

5/26: John and his younger son Adam are building a woodshed for us to store firewood. We are paying John; he has no work because of Covid. Edward shifts back and forth between rage and approval. He says it's a waste of money; we can use tarps to cover the wood. When I say John needs work, Edward says, "give him money." Seeing John build the shed, something he used to be able to do, upsets him. He recognizes his disability and hates it. A man wants to feel needed and capable.

5/31: There is an increase in Edward's emotional breakdowns of despair and angst. While I am vacuuming in the bedroom, he shouts a question. I may have been curt in answering. I stop the vacuum and go down to answer him, feeling the burden of the extra work that now falls to me. He is crying, saying, "I have nothing to live for anymore. I wish I could die. Why don't I die?!"

I try to give comfort. "Just go back to work," he says; "I'm a burden to you."

"No, you're not," I reply. Then I kiss him on the forehead and go back to work. When I finish vacuuming, I ask him to carry the vacuum downstairs for me. That seems to break through the despondent spell. He often says his life is a blank.

7/4: This is a difficult day. Early on, Edward cannot find his glasses. I had put them in the drawer where they are kept, and they were not there – two pairs. I am about to join a Zoom meditation intensive in five minutes, but I help him look. Finally, I find both pairs of glasses in the pocket of his shorts on the chair.

I say, "please keep them in the drawer." That is a mistake. He explodes, feeling I am ordering him around. He sits in the chair sulking.

"I wish I were dead," he says.

When there is a break in the Zoom class, I find him fixing tea without having showered or exercised, but I don't mention it. "Why didn't you put honey in my tea?" he asks, glaring at me.

"Because you didn't ask me to," I say.

He stays in a dark mood until late afternoon. Edward is ultra-sensitive to any perception of neglect. As his brain tissue erodes, karmic elements are in play for both of us – the old idea that he is not cared for and, for me, feeling under-appreciated. Both our needs are clashing. I must give love regardless of whether I get love in return. Edward needs me to give him unconditional love. This is a hard task. But maybe it is what I need to learn – humility and self-effacement, even under fire.

7/5: Dinner at our favorite restaurant, Garvan's. One of the best days in a long time. We reminisce about his army and Carnegie Mellon days, and our early romantic courtship. He is lively, gregarious, his old self. Long-term memories are often strong with people living with Alzheimer's. Even at home this intimacy continues. We lay naked in bed, each with a glass of wine, talking about our theatre days, and though he hasn't been able to have an erection for years, we fondle and make love in other ways.

12/9: I ask Edward to get some firewood. He takes the metal basket instead of the bag which I told him to use because the handle on the metal basket comes loose. When he comes in carrying lots of wood in the basket, the handle comes off, the wood spills, and we both get angry.

I say, "You yell at me a lot. I have a right to sometimes yell at you!" (In other words, I lost it).

Then we both get to the business of fixing the basket and calm down.

12/16: He can't find his phone. He's getting anxious. I say, "It's probably in the cubby under the wine rack where it's kept."

"Where is that?" he calls out. I get up from reading the newspaper and show him. The phone is there.

He yells and curses and blames me for bossing him around and causing him to be miserable. We sit down to talk. He wells up with self-pity. I comfort him by sitting close to him and holding his hand. I'm learning it is best not to say, "this is Alzheimer's."

"You treat me like a dog, an animal," he says defensively. "I want to die. There is no reason to go on."

I try to give him chores he can do – get more wood, chop up apples for applesauce, dry dishes – so that he feels useful, even if he is, as he says, "locked up in the house all the time."

When I try to bring him out of the gloom he says, "just leave me alone." So, I do. I let him mope and after a while he comes out of it and picks up the newspaper, holds it up close to his eyeglasses for a brief time, then just rests it on his lap.

2021

1/13: Impeachment hearings on TV all day. "What are you watching?" he asks. I tell him.

"Who's getting impeached?" It has been in the news all week.

"Do you know what's happening?" I ask.

He says, "no." It makes me sad that I can't share with him the news of the day.

I see him toying with the headphones. He is trying to adjust the volume and is frustrated. "A baby can do this," he says. "Show me again."

1/26: I ask Edward to help me fold laundry on the bed. I suggest he folds his stuff, and I fold mine. He says, "why don't you want to fold my laundry?" This is paranoia, the old idea surfacing that he is not cared for.

Later he sits by the fire sulking. I try to talk to him. "Shut up!" he yells. "I don't want to talk to you. Do you want me to leave?!" This is a threat he increasingly uses when he is angry. He stays in a funk all afternoon.

2/8: I wake Edward early to go for his eye exam at 10:00. "I don't like the way you treat me," he says. "Ordering me around like an animal, and it has to stop, now!" I don't reply. I know the paranoia overlays a frustrated lack of agency. He wants to do things himself but gets confused and needs my help, which he detests. At the eye doctor's I have to speak for him.

8/16: Edward goes out to the porch to meditate. When I come out, he is crying. He doesn't want me to touch him, but I do. I hug him and say it's okay to cry. "I feel useless; I have nothing to live for." He says this a lot.

I counter, "You have me, our family, the teaching. We're old; aging diminishes what we can do," I say. I don't mention Alzheimer's.

Earlier today I stubbed my pinkie toe badly and wrapped it. I am limping. "I have to keep my health," I say, "so I can care for you, the cats, and the house."

9/23: Two episodes of anger in two days lead me to suspect that the Memantine drug is losing its potency. In one episode, I set out Edward's lunch and tell him to just heat up the soup while I teach a Zoom class. When I come downstairs after the class, he is subdued and cool.

"How was your lunch?" I ask.

He says, "I wasn't hungry."

I find the lunch uneaten. I sense that he is angry and resentful because I was giving a class. I say this and he explodes with "f*ck you!" Then he admits what is bothering him. "You chose the class over me!" he says.

His hostility remains for hours. I must remember that he is acting out the disease. Later, having wine and cheese before supper, I relay to him what happened earlier. He doesn't remember anything.

2022

2/11: Edward forgets his morning routine. "It's your fault; you're always ordering me around," he says. He knows at a deeper level that he is losing control of his cognitive powers and must defend himself emotionally. His amygdala is activated to protect him from a perceived threat.

4/2: Edward gets annoyed if I tell him what to wear, yet he can also be sheepish and embarrassed. I get back from shopping and he is awake earlier than usual. He had put his flannel shirt on under his pajama top. He is having tea. When I remind him of his usual morning routine and suggest that he shower and just wear the flannel shirt without the pajama top he is deferential, eager to please. If I am sensitive to his sensitivity, and diplomatic, he will comply without saying, "you treat me like a baby."

***

In the interviews I held with Michael and David they reported a similar escalation in emotional outbursts of anger, frustration, and hostility. They spoke of their wives' inability to control emotional reactivity as the disease progressed into its later stages. Negative emotions were often projected onto others, including but not limited to themselves as caregivers. Michael said that there was a hostility period four years before Eileen's death in which she was often enraged. She routinely screamed at the bus driver. The caregiver, whom Michael had hired, quit. In our interview Michael described this difficult period:

I was sleeping in the back room when she began screaming in rage, yelling 'f*ck you' at me. I felt hatred, not for her but for the disease. I had to move out. I found *another apartment in the same building. We saw a psychopharmacologist who prescribed a medication: a big dose that was gradually reduced over a year. The rage disappeared into nothing.*

The medication stopped the rage, but the side effect was apathy. Around this time, Michael said that he had an accident. "I fell into a swimming pool and fractured my skull. I could no longer be the caregiver. Luckily, Medicaid gave us three years, 24/7 care," he said. "I would visit her every day."

David told me that when Karen's outbursts of rage got very bad, he relied on a close friend to help him defuse her moods.

He was my anchor. I could leave the house at that time, and I did. When I was home, if I was in a different room, Karen would get anxious looking for me. She lost the concept of time when I was out of sight. During the last twelve months of Karen's life, she occasionally got violent, out of frustration. She hit me. I had to maintain my cool. She'd get accusatory, insult me.

One day, while he was at the desk paying bills, Karen was pacing nearby. "She was anxious," David said:

Suddenly she gets a knife and comes toward me. I was the target. I picked up the phone and called 911. She heard me call and shouted, 'I do not have Alzheimer's!' When the police officers came, they took away the knife. She said to me 'I wish he [the policeman] would run me over.'

As the officers led Karen out to the police car to be hospitalized, she was saying, "I want to go back to my friends, my home. I miss my father." Medicare paid for

Karen's stay at the hospital's senior health unit for a month. When she returned home, she was under Hospice care. David told me that Karen said to him, "Oh, it's so good to be home." He was surprised and relieved because many times she wanted to go back to Westchester, to her family home.

Positive Actions and Preventive Measures

The role of caregiver is a learned role. In understanding and coping with Alzheimer's disease, I learned from my mistakes. Certain books, such as *The Thirty-Six Hour Day* by Mace and Rabins and Zeisel's *I'm Still Here*, helped to steer me in the right direction. They confirmed what I was discovering on my own and showed me creative ways to navigate the unknown path which Edward and I were traveling. Of particular importance is the reminder to the caregiver that the person in front of him or her is still a functioning human being with feelings and needs, regardless of the deterioration occurring in parts of the brain. Zeisel points to four emotional moods that begin to appear and grow when a person develops Alzheimer's disease. These moods are agitation, anxiety, apathy, and aggression. He calls them *the four As*. Spotting them and knowing how to lower their temperatures in practical ways becomes an art. As the disease progresses, abnormal behaviors, such as delusions and depression, are much harder to ameliorate. Zeisel concentrates on the four As, reminding the caregiver that when a person receives the news that he or she is now living with Alzheimer's disease, these moods are likely to appear as secondary consequences of the disease. They are not symptoms of the disease. Symptoms are caused by sickness in the brain – the abnormal growth of beta-amyloid and tau proteins that disrupt neural connections. As these proteins spread, wreaking havoc in the brain, symptoms appear. The first symptoms are damage to the temporal and parietal lobes. The hippocampus is especially affected, making retrieval of memories difficult. This results in the strange phenomenon of living in the present moment without access to what just happened (the past). As Wernicke and Broca speech areas are affected the person has difficulty finding the right words to express himself. He struggles to comprehend conversations. As neural connections at synapses deteriorate, the person living with Alzheimer's disease is unable to coordinate and perform sequences of actions. The proprioceptive function of knowing spatial configurations, including where one's body is in space, falters. All these, and other, symptoms are interrelated because the brain is a complex whole of interconnected neural circuits.

Pharmaceutical drugs, such as Aricept and Namenda, can slow down the physical process of decay for a time, but, so far, no cure is available. Zeisel contends that the four As are treatable by non-pharmaceutical methods. Treating these secondary consequences allows the person to live longer at a higher quality of life. Zeisel offers practical methods whereby the caregiver can make available to the person living with Alzheimer's disease this higher quality of life. As we alluded to in the chapter on nourishing the soul, Zeisel offers three major treatments. First, enhanced communication between the person and the caregiver can uncover pleasant, even joyful, memories from the person's life that he or she will enjoy talking about. When conversation is stimulated, the brain is exercised and the relationship between the person and the caregiver deepens, particularly when accompanied by sensory contact such as touch. A strong, loving relationship can soothe and lessen the fear and growing isolation that the person living with Alzheimer's disease feels. When Edward was encouraged to talk about his theatre days or his experiences in The School, his face would light up. He was reliving times when he felt happy and fulfilled.

Second, creating a calm, orderly, attractive environment reduces anxiety in the person living with Alzheimer's disease. When he or she is surrounded by familiar, meaningful objects, such as family photos or cherished art objects, he or she feels safe and relevant. Visits by family members add to the person's need to be recognized and appreciated. Our sons, their wives and children (four grandsons) were very supportive. Because they were educated in what to expect, they made Edward feel wanted and loved by their attentive presence. I remember a time at our condo in Florida, shortly before Edward was diagnosed with Alzheimer's disease, when he went to thrift stores and bought up large landscape paintings. Each painting featured a snow-capped mountain with water running down into a valley. We ended up with six such paintings covering the living room walls of the small condo. I asked him to take a few of them back; he refused. I only realized much later his objective in this compulsive undertaking. He was surrounding himself with reminders of the spiritual work to which his life was dedicated. The mountain was the Himalaya, the refuge of sannyasins, present and past, whose singular aim in life was Self-realization.

Thirdly, the caregiver can help bring joy and a sense of accomplishment to the person living with Alzheimer's disease if he or she taps into and uncovers the person's creative interests. Each day becomes enlivened with practical activities that feed the person's self-esteem, while simultaneously strengthening the relationship between the person and the caregiver. The healing, invigorating energy of engaging a person's creativity was observed in Edward's Japanese brush painting efforts, Eileen's love of music, and Karen and David's art collaboration.

Below is a bullet list of positive actions the caregiver can take to help his or her loved one who is living with Alzheimer's disease. Some suggestions may overlap those already laid out in previous chapters. Also included are preventive measures which are valuable lifestyle actions. These measures help not only the person living with Alzheimer's disease but also anyone who is trying to optimize his or her health and thus avoid the possible onset of dementia. Since only 2 per cent of people who contract Alzheimer's disease have a genetic propensity, the other 98 per cent can choose a lifestyle that promotes neurological health.

- Establish a daily routine of ordinary actions like showering, dressing, eating, et cetera. Repetition reinforces the neural connections necessary for the sequencing of actions.
- Include in the routine brisk walking, preferably outside in the natural world. Physical exercise, both aerobic and simple walking, stimulates neural connections and is shown to reduce the risk of contracting dementia. When walking, vary the places and routes; staying with what is familiar encourages the brain to just vegetate on automatic pilot.
- When giving directions for any work or activity, keep it simple; one action at a time. The sequence will tie

itself together as you move along.

- Practice presence yourself and encourage your loved one to do the same. Mindfulness calms and energizes the brain in positive ways.

- Do things together, both fun and serious. Especially important is some type of regular meditation or contemplative prayer, preferably shared. The engagement of attention that meditation requires and the serenity that it can produce, even if temporary, nourish the prefrontal cortex and relax the whole brain. The mind-body continuum supports the inclusion of both physical and mental-emotional-spiritual exercise for holistic health.

- Diet is important. One dietary regimen that geriatricians and other doctors recommend is the Mediterranean diet that includes fresh, local, and seasonal vegetables and fruits. Although the food may cost more, it is advisable to buy organic to avoid pesticides. B vitamins, such as folic acid, vitamins D and E have been shown to enhance brain health including memory.

- Go easy on or abstain from alcoholic beverages. There is a connection between misuse of alcohol and dementia.

- A good night's sleep is important – seven to nine hours preferably – for brain health. During sleep, the information of the day is digested. The glial cells busily clean the brain so that beta-amyloid and tau proteins don't accumulate. If sleep apnea develops, get it treated.

- Give clues and props to stimulate but not test the loved one's memory; avoid saying things like "don't you remember….?"

- Lay out his clothes because he won't remember which dresser drawers contain which clothing. Let him dress himself. Wait patiently (but not obtrusively) for him to finish. Only help if he gets agitated and frustrated.

- Keep a sense of humor and lightness of tone, especially at times when he doesn't remember something and gets frustrated. Connect with a smile.

- Examine the house to be sure that navigation between rooms is as easy as possible. Remove furniture that might invite a fall. Eliminate steps if possible. I removed an ottoman in front of the wing-back chair where Edward often sat so that he could walk away from the chair safely. As the disease progressed, his balance was affected, so when he stood up, I started a routine where we marched in place to exercise his legs and regain balance before he started to walk. Eventually he needed a walker.

- In the bathroom, put up grab bars wherever they are needed. Our older son, John, who is a master carpenter, installed high quality grab bars in the shower area and by the toilet, so that Edward could exit the bathtub safely and stand up in a balanced way after using the toilet.

- Create a peaceful atmosphere in the house by playing calming music. Buy fresh flowers for the dinner table. Light a candle to make the meal special.

- Evenings can be rough because of the sundown syndrome, especially as the disease progresses. Find ways to measure the day's activities so that your loved one is not overtired by evening. It is important to go out together and do things, like grocery shopping, for example. But any prolonged or excessive changes in the environment can produce stress, disorientation, and fear. Fatigue can trigger anxiety and sometimes aggressive remarks.

- When laying out food on dinner plates, separate the items and discreetly tell him what they are. If he wants to mix and mash the items, let him. Don't say "that's not the way to eat." The less one 'corrects' the person living with

Alzheimer's, the better. I learned the hard way to keep quiet and let be.

- Pets are wonderful companions. So long as you feed them, a dog or cat only wants to give you love. Hospice offers pet care for terminal patients enrolled in their program. They also offer live music by people, such as professional violinists, who volunteer their services. Edward and our orange cat, Henry, were inseparable buddies. Until the last days when Edward became weak, incoherent, and bedridden, Henry would always find Edward's lap. Together they meditated or just sat quietly in perfect communion.

- Be sure to get help from family and friends so that stress does not build up over time and erode your health as caregiver. An afternoon out, confident that your loved one is safe and cared for, refreshes mind-body and spirit.

Our lives have a beginning and an ending. In between, we don't think much about the finality that will come. Because of the human ability to be aware of death, as part of the gift of life, recognition of finality lodges somewhere in a dark corner of the mind, until a time arrives when it comes to the light and confronts us. As we now reach the last chapter of our inquiry into Alzheimer's disease, we will review, largely through journal entries, the final year of Edward's life. Everything that is final – whether it be the final year of high school, graduation from college, retirement from a satisfying career, the end of reproductive life, and finally death of the body – deserves our respectful observance and our gratitude for all that came before.

Chapter Seven: **The Final Year**

In the book *Living with Alzheimer's and Other Dementias,* an essay is included by a granddaughter who recalls the last days of her grandmother's life. The elderly woman had Alzheimer's disease. She had long entertained the delusion that her son was her husband, and that her daughter-in-law had taken him away from her. The animosity between the two women had solidified. The granddaughter relates that on her deathbed her grandmother held the hand of her daughter-in-law. Although the grandmother could no longer speak, she was able to understand everything that was said to her, including the true facts about her son and his wife. She knew the unreality of the delusion and grasped the hand of the daughter-in-law in love.

This story illustrates the persistence in our life, and at our death, of underlying awareness. The life-death cycle is a whole, pervaded by awareness. Conscious awareness never leaves us because it is us. David told me that when Karen came home from the hospital, after the violent incident with the knife, she calmed down and was happy to be home. She qualified for Hospice care. "After a couple of weeks at home," he related, "she didn't want to get up from bed. She didn't want to eat. The Hospice nurse said she was now terminal. I believe she had decided to die at home." David went on to describe Karen's last days:

There was awareness on some level, and she made a choice. I provided fluids. She was on morphine. The Hospice nurse kept her comfortable and clean. I was sleeping on the couch. Her breaths became labored. Then early on the morning of September 10th, 2021, I couldn't hear her breathing. Her eyes were closed. To witness her death was the most profound experience of my life. I sat with her in the morning light, the golden light. Our stepson and her close friend were with me. I felt her presence as she dropped the body.[92]

Michael recalls that during the last month of Eileen's life there was no pain, except for bed sores. She was bedridden and was lifted to a chair only to eat. "She couldn't talk months before, but sometimes she sang with me," he said. "When I was with her, I felt love and sadness. What she taught me came from love. Before she was sick, I was going through a difficult work situation. I had financial worries. We were in bed. I woke her to ask if everything will be alright. 'No,' she said, 'everything *is* alright.'" In describing his wife's last days Michael said:

In the end she was lying there, a lump. I saw death in her face, yet she was aware, because when I lay next to her, she clasped my thumb. Then when our friends came over we meditated as she lay still, her eyes closed. Eileen was in that envelope of absolute stillness. When the Hospice chaplain entered the room, she said it was like walking into a holy temple. When Eileen was gone, I stayed with her body and sang. I heard that pieces of the person, like hearing, live on briefly. The people from the funeral home took her body away in a bag. Later, when I was at the computer, writing out the funeral list, I felt her presence standing behind me.[93]

I asked Reverend Diane what she has witnessed regarding the death of the body and whether her dying patients believed in a soul. She said:

I have watched many deaths. There are different

answers from everyone. I believe there is a spark of the divine in each of us, the soul, deeply connected to our intuition, our heart. I see a connection to the divine in my patients, even at the last breath which may be peaceful or agitated. Even with Alzheimer's, the spark is still there; the light is still there. The brain is overrated. There's more than just the brain. At the end, systems shut down, but chemicals are released to hold on to life. The person may suddenly sit up and eat, then die. The source is always there. The body fails us. The soul is unaffected by the body-mind condition. When the body takes its last breath there's a silence, a stillness that is sacred. The soul may take time to remove itself from the container – the rental unit I call it – to completely let go and move on. Even if someone cannot speak, the spark is still there. It leaves when the brain has stopped.[94]

In 2022, about a year before Edward's death, two main incidents accelerated the progression of the disease: a one-month vacation in Florida in February-March and, in October, a move to a one-story ranch. The move was the more influential event. It triggered episodes of severe delusion, depression, and frenetic behavior which required medication. Edward's doctor prescribed an anti-psychotic drug, Haloperidol (Haldol). Edward stayed on the drug for about two weeks, after which he stopped taking it because the reaction to the move was subsiding. The doctor and I also thought it best if Edward stopped drinking wine, though he had never had more than a half-glass at dinner. He did not resist this new abstinence. He stopped taking Memantine as it was no longer working.

Journal entries

The following journal entries trace Edward's final year.

They show the chronological progression of the disease. During these months I felt a crescendo, as if we were living a musical composition that increased in tempo and volume towards a finale. Episodes of delusion and depression multiplied. Several entries show Capgras delusion. In this type of delusion, the person who is seen, whose face is very familiar, is not recognized. He or she is believed to be an imposter. The throughline of denial, the fortress Edward's mind had created to sustain sanity, began to crumble under the weight of the evidence that the disease was destroying his brain. Awareness alerted him that he could no longer dismiss the strange symptoms he was experiencing as the product of normal aging. There was fear, but also glimpses of acceptance. The acknowledgement of the arrival of death was only eased at times by the spiritual belief, which we shared, that 'I am not this sickness; I am not this body.' Flashes of normalcy, clarity, and even insight are interwoven with acute experiences of morbidity, hallucinations of an alternate reality, and mental chaos. I have no doubt that the vacation to Florida and particularly the move to the new house exacerbated his condition. I bear some responsibility for this aggravation of his symptoms since I initiated the decision to move. Rationalizing that the disease would have advanced anyway gives me little solace.

In the final stage of Alzheimer's disease, there are hard lessons to be learned. Learning how to engage with but also submit to a terminal illness, especially the kind that kills the brain, is a daily task for the loved one and the caregiver. Yielding to circumstances, as they are, is a strength, not a weakness. If the heart can remain compassionate and loving, then even though there is physical illness and dissolution, there is emotional-spiritual health.

April 2022 - March 2023

4/21: We are watching TV. Out of the blue Edward asks, "where is the key?"

"What key?" I reply.

"The key to the door," he says.

"What door?" I ask.

"I don't know; the key I gave you," he says.

"This is your imagination," I say. I feel bewildered. We are in two separate worlds.

5/5: Bizarre bowel movement episode. While I am conducting a Zoom class, I hear Edward come downstairs and go into the bathroom. I hear him mumbling angrily and see him at the base of the steps, naked. I need to finish the class but all the while I am worried. Why is he naked? Where is he now? I can hardly concentrate on what I am teaching. After the class, I find him upstairs lying on the bed. There are smeared feces on the front of his undershirt and briefs. He says that I came in from outside with a five-foot stick and gave it to him, and I was to blame for the poop. Even as he speaks, I see bafflement and fear in his eyes. I feel so unprepared for this. When I say, "you're fantasizing; Alzheimer's can do that," he flinches and says, "stop that Alzheimer's stuff – it's you!" I back away from the bed and wait. When he calms down, I say, "let's go downstairs and clean you up." As I pick up the soiled clothes that he left on a chair, I take a moment to inspect the chair to see if there are feces on it; I don't see any. In the downstairs bathroom, I help him clean himself. While he takes a shower, I take his clothes to the laundry sink, turn the hot water on, and wash out the poop. The smell reminds me of washing out soiled baby onesies, but I feel nauseous rather than neutral because this isn't normal. When he is out of the shower and changed into fresh clothes, we sit on the terrace and discuss what happened. He appears calm and reasonable. I feel anxious about what might be a new stage in the disease, but when I look over at him a warmth rises in me. This man was once my debonair lover, my partner in putting on plays at the Rhode Island summer stock company he created. I am remembering how we worked hard rehearsing and performing during the day and evening, then made love on the beach at night. We were young, carefree, healthy.

Edward begins this important conversation.

"A new stage," he says. "I am sorry for you. Tell me the truth, am I going batty?"

"It's Alzheimer's," I say softly, "and the fantasizing about the stick shows brain tissue deterioration, perhaps on the right hemisphere where creative ideas are formed."

He seems to accept this.

"It is important not to deny it," he says, "but just live through it. I am not afraid."

"But upstairs in the dream state you were confused and projected it onto me," I say. "It's natural to defend yourself from the unknown." He nods in agreement.

"You are cogent right now and we can speak reasonably," I say.

"Yes," he says. "I hope I can remember who I am, that knowing my identity doesn't go as my memory goes. We have studied and practiced the teaching for many years."

"It's my job to remind you of who you are," I offer, "especially when you are in this imagined reality."

We don't talk about the bowel incontinence, but I say, quietly, "perhaps you should wear a Depends." He says nothing to that. Later, watching TV in the den, he asks me who is watching TV upstairs. I say we don't have a TV upstairs; there's just us here.

5/6: "When are we going back?" he asks. He thinks we are in Florida. Then he quickly checks himself and says, "we're not going back, are we. We are back." He is aware.

5/10: Second bowel movement incident.

"I stood up and it popped out of me," Edward says. "You did this. You were standing by the bathroom door and did this to me. You f*cked me up."

"No, this came from your body," I say softly.

"It's my brain, right?" he says, agitated, pointing to his head.

I nod. I think he feels as if he is regressing into infancy.

5/11: Edward says he won't wear Depends. I put a Depend next to his underwear for when he gets out of the shower. He hides it in his drawer and doesn't put it on under his briefs.

5/16: We go to the doctor for a rectal exam; it shows a loose sphincter muscle and enlarged prostate. There may be damaged nerve connections to the involuntary sphincter muscle.

5/18: Before bed I say, "do you want me to turn off the TV for you?"

He says, "maybe somebody else wants it on."

"There's only you and me here," I say.

"Well, there was somebody in the shower," he says. I don't reply. What good would it do?

As the delusions increase, I am getting more alarmed. I don't want to call my sons and alarm them, yet I wish I could confide in someone. My daughter-in-law Magda thinks I should hire a helper.

6/4: After watching a movie we are in bed and Edward says, "I guess our guest slipped out after the movie."

"What guest?" I query.

"I must have been dreaming," he says, laughing.

6/5: There were three episodes of fantasizing today:

1) "Ludge took away my car and driver's license along with the lady eye doctor," he says, petulantly.

2) Driving home from a walk on the rail trail, the car in front of us turns and he says, "is that our car? He was following us."

3) We are putting shoes on to take the cats out for a walk when he says, "I don't even have a family and kids, and I should. I have nothing."

"I am your wife and you have two grown sons. Did you forget?" I ask.

"Yes, I did," he says, without anger. He *can* come back

to reality from fantasy.

6/6: As I am about to get in the shower he asks, "where do I sleep tonight?" I point to our bed. "Right," he says. "I just wanted to make sure." He is aware. He's covering up.

6/8: Edward asks, for the umpteenth time, "are we married?"

"Yes, fifty-four years," I say.

"I'm forgetting larger spans of time," he says. "I go over the houses we lived in starting with East 9th St."

"Then you remember these houses?" I ask.

"No," he says, "my brain is going. It's shocking. What's happening to me?"

"Alzheimer's," I say. He looks at me as if hearing this for the first time.

6/17: We are using Vaseline to help heal the sore on Edward's cheek. He puts it on his hair, thinking it is mousse! He tries to poop five or six times a day. It's becoming compulsive. He fears another accident. So do I.

6/19: Moments of awareness and lucidity. It is Father's Day. We have a party at our house. We watch a one-hour interview of Jean Klein, a spiritual teacher whose books Edward has read several times. Our grandson Mark converted the interview from VHS to DVD as a present to his grandfather. Edward follows it well. The interview is slow enough for him to follow the conversation. He is riveted, his attention full. His face lights up. Afterwards, Edward speaks of the interview with ardor and clarity. "It reminds me of what is true that I knew," he says. "The teaching is pure, everything else in my mind is weakened, but I feel purified."

6/22: Having lunch at a favorite café:

"My brain feels dull," he says.

"A blank?" I ask.

"Yes, but a conscious blank."

"You mean you're aware of it?" I ask.

"Yes. I look out here and I feel the past, that we've been here before, but memories, thoughts about what I see, don't come; memories don't come."

"Just a feeling?" I ask.

"Yes," he says, nodding.

Feelings, which are related to intuition and instinct, are still functional in his brain. I am relieved to see that there is still a strong perceptiveness and reflective functioning. He is able to express this difference between thoughts and feelings. In recent days, I notice moments of clarity and awareness juxtaposed to episodes of forgetting and fantasizing. I pray that the moments of clarity persist, but I worry that they will diminish.

6/23: I come home from shopping and hear water running. I find water running full blast in the bathroom sink. Edward is lying in bed awake. He says he didn't hear the water. "It's your fault," he says. "You harass me. I'm moving out!" I know this projection is not him, but I still feel the sting of his attack in my gut. After meditation he calms down. Edward is worried again about money. He fantasizes about being cheated by the franchisee of the

IHOP we own. I reassure him that everything is fine financially.

6/27: The mix of delusion and awareness has me wondering if he is moving into a more severe stage of Alzheimer's disease.

After meditation he says, "I'm not comfortable with this situation we are in."

"What situation?" I ask, thinking that he is talking about the move that we are considering.

"Our illegal relationship," he says. "We're not married."

"Yes, we are. Fifty-four years," I say, as I hear my voice harden with impatience. I know I need to be patient, but I am tired of hearing him say this. How many times do I give the same answer, and he still asks.

"My brain is scrambled," he says. He is quiet a moment, then he says, "I see that I go into another reality and get stuck in it. Can you help me with this?"

His admission of need, and the meekness accompanying it, dissolves my impatience. "I am here for you always," I say, "throughout Alzheimer's."

"I don't want to drag you into this," he says.

"I'm with you," I say. "We are in this together. I am aware of what is happening to you; I am here to help. Remember, it's all a dream – *maya*, the world is an illusion."

"Yes, but I'm in a dream within a dream," he says, "and that's not allowed."

I am struck by the split screen of his awareness of his condition and the ability sometimes to talk about it, in contrast to cognitive decline. I witness this decay, and sometimes he does. Before bed Edward says, "Who was that person that I escorted into the house today?"

"You're imagining a scene that didn't happen," I say.

6/28: In bed, before sleep, Edward says, "did I sign the paper that that man brought for me to join the service?"

"There was no paper," I say. Edward served in the army. He is mixing up that memory with fantasy. "You mean the army?" I ask.

"Yes, they come to get you," he says.

I play along. "You're too old," I say.

"They work their way up," he says, frowning. I smile.

6/30: Edward asks again about money and whether we are married. I answer straightforwardly. This is becoming routine. He dozes during the day. At night he sleeps twelve to thirteen hours. Is this a sign that the disease is spreading?

7/3: We are invited to have lunch at the house of our good friends, Diane and Earl. They live on the retreat property of The School of Practical Philosophy in Wallkill, NY. Other people who are, or were, in The School are also invited. Before we leave, Donald, a School colleague who learned woodworking from Edward, takes us on a golf cart to see recent improvements to the property. This 'tour' affects Edward, stirring his memory. On the way home he speaks of his experience in The School and its great effect on him.

"I think there is a hierarchy of true being, levels of refinement," he says. "I have a fuzzy feeling in my stomach."

"Is it the food?" I ask.

"No, no; being at the property I was remembering many years of commitment and involvement. So now I have mixed emotions. I am depressed but also feeling fortunate to re-experience those times."

This was a high level of expression of something dear to Edward. I feel happy for him. Just being in the place where he gave himself to the study of spiritual teachings elicited memories that were solid and heartfelt. Often, before we go to sleep, he gets maudlin, even mean, cursing about the futility of his life, blaming me sometimes and threatening to leave. Not tonight.

7/14: Edward doesn't know who I am.

"I'm going to rent a house and live by myself, have some privacy," he says. I tell him I am his wife and that his plan won't work unless I go too.

"This is distressing," I say, "forgetting who I am."

He puts his hand on mine. I see recognition in his eyes. "I can't help it," he says.

"I know," I say.

7/17: Edward sleeps more during the day. He can only read the headlines of the paper since they are in large print. He doesn't study his spiritual material. I start reading aloud to him from one of our spiritual books, every day.

7/23: Out on the terrace Edward again doesn't believe I

am his wife.

"Where is my family!?" he says, frantically. "If I'm sick and if my brain is cuckoo, then I want to die."

He is still partly denying Alzheimer's and partly admitting it. At dinner he admits he was pretending that he didn't have Alzheimer's.

"I had to protect myself," he says. "I am concerned about you as I get worse. What about you?" he asks.

"We are married," I reply. "We're a team. We took vows."

7/27: Getting up in the morning he asks, "are you my sister?"

"No, your wife," I answer.

"How long?" he asks.

"Fifty-four years," I say.

He laughs, then gets morose. "I've had a useless life."

"No, a useful life." I give examples. They seem to register.

"Thanks for getting me out of the doldrums," he says.

8/7: A mix of anger, paranoia, and awareness today.

"I'm in a f*ckin' prison here. Where's my car? I can drive! You took it!" He begins to cry. "I don't want to live anymore. I should kill myself."

I embrace him, remind him of those who care about him.

I find out I have Covid. I tell Edward. He gets anxious about himself. Everything always reverts to him. This makes me angry and I'm about to tell him he is being selfish. Then I remember, he can't help it.

"I want out of here. Where is the key to my car?!" he shouts.

He is 'f*cking' this and that, so I leave the room. I go into the bedroom, close the door, and sit down. I take some deep breaths. Stay mindful, I tell myself. Then I start to cry.

At 8:30 pm we have a crystal-clear conversation about what is happening to his brain. I tell him that he just had a delusionary experience about a man coming to the house to steal our car. He asks me four times where our car is, and I show him four times. He is close to tears.

"I will never, never harm you," he says. "I can't believe this is happening to me. I'm going crazy."

We speak about how there are clear moments, like now, and imaginary ones. "Was I gruff?" he asks, remorsefully.

"Yes, but I can deal with that now. I love you."

"I love you too," he says. "I feel that this is a breakthrough day, that I see and have to accept what is happening to me." He sees the delusion about the car. Even as he keeps asking about the car, he can at the same time witness the delusion that his brain concocts. "Are you scared of me? I don't want you to be scared of me," he says.

"No, I'm not scared. I know you. We need to accept what's happening to you." He nods in agreement. Is this the day of true acceptance?

8/17: The disconnect from reality is growing. We call Edward's sister Dolores. Later, he says, "I'm glad she came." He thinks Dolores came to visit us, but it was a phone call.

"Who is taking care of me?" he asks.

"I am," I say. In the moment he clearly realizes he needs care.

9/8: Edward keeps talking about his mother.

"Where is Mum? She was right here," he says.

"You are imagining this," I say.

"Forget it; we're talking about something that didn't happen," he says. So, after the fact he knows that he imagined something, but the imagined reality rose up first, out of his control.

9/17: Delusions before bed:

"What am I doing here? Someone keeps stealing my car. I'm single," he says.

"No, we are married," I reply. I look at him and speak slowly. "We have two sons, John and James."

"No, John is gone," he says.

"No, he just turned fifty," I say. "You confuse him with your brother Ludge who died."

He considers this. "I feel lost," he says, "no past or future. Just the present."

9/18: Two days in a row, Edward sits for hours organizing the contents of his night table drawer. It's obsessive-compulsive. He says he is arranging his 'wallets'. As neural networks in the brain become less connected, perhaps organizing contents of a drawer is analogous to ordering the mind.

9/20: Edward is in a bad mood. He sits sullen, isolated. I try to rouse him. He looks at me with dagger eyes, as if to blame me, then says, "I'm going crazy, that's all!"

9/22: He is organizing the contents of his drawer again. "I've got so many wallets," he says. Edward mistakes eyeglass cases and a small pad for wallets. In bed at night, he awakens suddenly, frightened. "How can this be happening to me?" he asks. "What did I do to deserve this? What sin did I commit? All my past, my experience, is gone. I can't remember us, our marriage, our life together."

Listening to him is heartbreaking. I hug him close and say, "but at least you are aware of this loss of memory." I feel his rib bones through the bed clothes. He is losing weight. My eyes brim with tears. I am remembering a body that is vigorous, strong, and beautiful.

"But it will get worse," he says. "I don't want to live like this."

"It's up to God what happens in our old age." I say. "Everyone has infirmities. We have each other. I will help you." In some ways these periods of awakening are more painful for him than the pitiful repetitions of organizing his 'wallets'.

9/27: Edward opens the freezer to get a popsicle. He thinks the rectangular blue ice pack is a popsicle. We are packing up to move. With boxes everywhere this chaos may accentuate his confusion. "You moved papers from my drawer," he says, "information that I need to make this deal, could make us a lot of money, all blown up! I'll have to get the information again!"

10/8: The move happens. It accelerates symptoms, magnifies existing ones, and produces new ones. I expected a difficult transition, but Edward's behavior is becoming psychotic. He asks, over and over, "where am I?" and "how much money do we have? Where is it?". In one episode he accuses me, saying, "you are evil, you want my money!" He opens the side door of the house and starts walking up the street to "go home and get away from you!" I walk after him to stop him. He turns and raises his fist. "I'll punch you in the face," he shouts. I back off and call James to come over and help get his dad back into the house. This is the first time I have been afraid of Edward. I wish we hadn't moved. I blame myself for making this decision. It has made the situation worse. Later that night while sleeping, in a dream state, he murmurs, "I was very angry, and my fists were swinging," as if to say he knew he had almost done something he would regret.

Awareness of his condition emerges like switching on a light and we can talk about it. Then he reverts into darkness. "How can you stand being with me, putting up with this?" he says.

"In sickness and in health," I say.

"I am glad I have you to take care of me," he replies.

10/9: We are unpacking at the new house; it's around 5:00 pm. Edward is helping me put some garden items in the barn. His mood suddenly changes and with an accusatory tone he says, "something is fishy, I want to know what's going on!" I tell him to go inside and rest, that I will finish up. When I go back inside he is sitting on the couch, dagger eyes. He accuses me of bringing him here against his will. "You kidnapped me!" he says. I try to calm him. When I bring him a cup of mint tea, to relax him, he says, "I won't drink it. You spiked it!" I call John; I hand the phone to Edward. John tries to bring his dad back to reality. He succeeds somewhat. Edward apologizes to me, but I cannot trust him. I have never felt this way about Edward. He was always trustworthy. He can't believe what he said to me and promises to do his best to "handle" it and stay aware. He admits he was defending himself against an illusory attack. He even admits his sickness. When dressing for bed, he reverts to fantasy. He can't control his mood swings. The amygdala has free rein.

"You aren't my wife," he says. "Don't get close. I'm single. I've been in Florida for a while and I'm going back."

"You are fantasizing again," I say.

"I don't believe you," he says, running his hands through his hair. I leave him as he gets into bed, but then I hear him rummaging around. He takes his wallet from the bedside drawer and hides it with him in bed.

10/13: For three hours midday Edward is in an alternate reality: delusionary and paranoid. He says he needs to go to Florida to live in a residence in the IHOP. I am not his wife; he has a wife named Lyla. He needs his car, and someone told him he had to go down to Florida because his business is jeopardized. He is very agitated. I try to stay calm, but I feel my insides churning with anxiety. He says

245

it was his friend Martin who told him there was something suspicious going on with the IHOP. "Martin died two years ago," I say. He is shocked.

10/15: Edward is fixated on his wallet. He is organizing items in his bedside drawer again. We go shopping. He thinks we went to the movies too. When it is bedtime, he gets in bed on my side. When I come to bed and ask him to move over he says, "get out, you son of a bitch!" He never used that word before.

"You'll never be in this bed with me!" he shouts.

"But I'm your wife," I say.

"No, you're not and never will be," he says. He gets out of bed, takes his clothes to the living room, and begins to change into them. When I try to tell him again that I am his wife, he says "No, you're not. A man just came into my bedroom, tried to put the make on me."

"That was me," I say. I feel like I am talking to a stranger.

"I don't trust this house," he says. "There are people here."

10/21: Back and forth from normalcy to fantasy. I call Edward's doctor. He suggests Haldol, an anti-psychotic drug that should calm Edward's agitation. He starts taking it. He says it makes him feel "strange, drugged" but it hasn't stopped the hallucinations. "You kidnapped me," he says. "That woman..." (pointing to me) "...is not my wife." Last night, he hid his wallet in his sock, and said he couldn't find it. We looked everywhere. Then I saw a bulge in his sock. He knew it was there all the time. There is craftiness in his madness. He says he hid it so "no one will get my money." I call John again to ask him to talk his dad down. This is so burdensome for the boys, but I rely on them. I need their help. I feel totally unequipped to deal with this horror.

10/24-26: Three days without incident. He still hallucinates but without vitriol, just mystified confusion.

"You are my wife, really?" he asks. "My wife is Lyla Yastion," he says.

"That's who I am," I say. "Don't I look like her?"

"Yes, you do!" he says.

He doesn't drink wine now. I read that the combination of Haldol and alcohol can cause a rise in aggression and other negative emotions. Haldol can also, as a side effect, induce hallucinations.

11/24: Deterioration of posture, slumping, slow shuffle; Edward is very thin. He forgets where rooms are in the house. He has trouble reaching for a knob to a drawer or placing a teacup on a coaster. This lack of motor coordination may involve deteriorating eyesight. He loses touch with where his body is in space.

11/26: There is a meditation intensive at a nearby ashram. I ask Edward if he feels up to it. He says, "Sure, remember, I'm a spiritual being." We go to the intensive. It is a very supportive, loving atmosphere. Gurudev's theme for the day is gratitude. He says, "sacrifice the ego and align yourself with the universe." At the end of the intensive, darshan is offered. This is a ritual in which a devotee bows in front of the guru, meets his eyes, and asks for guidance. I ask for Gurudev's help to care for my husband with a pure heart. Although Edward dozed off and on during the intensive, he was able to stay in the good company of the ashram for the whole day. By osmosis he was helped.

12/3: Edward's niece, Christina, and her husband, Donald, are visiting. We hold a Christmas party in their honor. At the party, Edward conducts a phenomenal philosophy class. As we gather in the living room after supper, he emerges from a stupor-like nap, and, sitting in his wing-back chair, for twenty minutes holds his 'students' spellbound. His manner is normal, his speech and sequencing of thought and expression lucid, and at times even brilliant. There is an ease and light touch in his delivery that harkens back to the classes he tutored at The School.

12/14: Edward stops taking Haldol. I hoped that the medication would stop the hallucinations. It didn't, and side effects are stiffness and muscular weakness. These effects could lead to falls. His growing familiarity with the new house is eliminating the paranoid episodes.

12/17: We go to the theatre in Poughkeepsie to hear Handel's *Messiah*, then out to dinner. On our way home, we stop at a strip mall to get a few groceries. Edward is tired. He doesn't want to come in with me, so I leave him in the car and walk quickly into the supermarket. When I return, he is not in the car. I see him walking up towards the cinema. I catch up with him. Edward is disoriented. He thinks he is walking to our house. He fantasizes about having "no money for the meter and it is necessary to have a meeting of the board to sort out and put in order the situation," he says. There is no board, but there is a situation.

This is a wake-up call for me as his caregiver: don't leave him unattended. I thank God that I saw him before he disappeared. I would have had to call the police. I feel so guilty that I left him in the car. What was I thinking?

12/21: Edward sleeps seventeen hours straight. He talks in his sleep, asking me if it is time to meditate. Several times he says the dedication and then, "my hands are folded on my chest, ready to meditate." It is touching to hear this. I feel myself starting to cry. I am witnessing how the inner strength of a person, what matters most to him, remains strong in consciousness.

12/23: Edward's eyes look vacant and cloudy. He touches things to locate them rather than seeing them. He doesn't make eye contact. John, who is visiting, notices this.

12/24: Edward falls this evening in the living room for the second time. He gets off balance when he stands. His leg muscles are getting weak. When he fell he rolled on the rug, coming within inches of the stone fireplace ledge with his head. Luckily, when we moved here, John covered the sharp edge with a rubber gasket. I have removed the ottoman and coffee table. I am teaching Edward to bounce his knees and then march in place every time he stands up, but he forgets if I'm not there. We march around the house.

1/1/2023: It is the new year. The confusion starts at supper. He thinks he is not in America. He is fearful.

"Of what?" I ask.

"Of whatever comes next," he says.

"There is nothing to fear," I say. "This is our home."

Later, after watching a segment about obesity on *60 Minutes*, his favorite program, he says there are people in the living room with equipment and drugs, for weight loss. Though he is lean he is identifying himself with the content of the TV segment. He is obsessed with this hallucination. I tell him it is just a TV program, not about him. He says, "there is something wrong with my brain." Something in his brain is watching the scene he is creating inside his brain.

1/2: Edward is losing interest in TV, news, and football. He asks me before he showers, "what is that?" pointing to the towel. "And that?" he asks, pointing to the floor mat. His inability to recognize objects signals damage to the inferotemporal cortex (IT).

1/7: I put the toothpaste on Edward's toothbrush; otherwise, when he tries to do it, the toothpaste spills into the sink.

1/8: At meals there's minimal conversation. When I mention this, Edward tries to converse, but his speech is faltering, disjointed. I ask him how he feels. He says, "confused; I've been confused for six months." As I am fixing supper, he comes into the kitchen from watching TV and asks, "are you still up?" He is losing a sense of linear time.

1/13: At breakfast, Edward slurps cereal as if it were soup. After we eat, he sits on the sofa and listens to the CDs I put on in the morning. When I come in to join him, he asks, "where are the festivities?"

"What festivities?" I ask.

"The marriages," he says.

"Of whom?" I ask.

"Our younger son, John."

"You mean James. He's been married twenty-one years," I say.

"It's not festive here," he says, disappointed.

I help him dress in the morning and evening now – a further stage in the disease. I turn on and adjust the shower in the morning. He asks me, "what do I do in here?"

"Wash your body," I say.

"Do I use soap? Wash my whole body?" he asks.

I demonstrate what he is to do. John has put up grab bars in the shower area and in front of the toilet. Tonight, as Edward sleeps, a pattern seems to be forming – lots of twitching, moving his legs, talking out loud. At times he is breathless as if he is in a war zone. At about 5:00 am, I snuggle against his back to calm him. Even as I feel my body against his, I feel our separateness. He is lost in a disease that, like a demon, will not let go of him. I cannot rescue him. This stark fact fills me with sorrow.

1/14: We argue about the toilet being clogged – again. He uses too much paper. I get the plunger, upset.

"You do it this time!" I say.

He resists at first but then complies, saying, "this is the end of our relationship!"

"The alternative is a nursing home," I counter, angry and fed up.

He becomes subdued but I immediately regret the threat. I leave the bathroom to stew in private. After a few minutes of self-pity, I relax the tension in my shoulders, close my eyes, and meditate.

1/20: At dinner he says, "what's in this dish?"

"Grapes," I say. He begins to put salad on top of his cornbread.

2/1: Edward's eighty-ninth birthday. I bake his favorite cake. This makes him happy.

2/9: Appointment with a geriatrician, Dr. Jodi Friedman. Edward has an interview, then an evaluation using a verbal test. He answers eight out of thirty questions and draws a clock that looks like an amoeba. Dr. Friedman thinks he should have an echocardiogram because of a heart murmur.

2/21: Edward is eating less and less. He's skinny; his rib bones show. It's like the flesh is shrinking. He sleeps long hours. He still talks in his sleep. It's getting harder for him to comprehend speech. I speak slower and louder. Broca's area in the brain is damaged.

2/23: "When do people usually die?" Edward asks. "It varies," I say.

2/24: During evening meditation, which we always practice together, he is making lots of sounds with his mouth and nose, sucking sounds and sniffing. He keeps moving his feet. Midway into the meditation, he asks, "what are we waiting for?" and then "we just drove into the garage." When I ask if he can put his attention on the mantra he says, "yes, but I don't know for how long." He hasn't pooped in two days, and he has a stomachache. Before bed I give him Alka seltzer and put a heating pad on his stomach. He isn't eating much. He says he just wants to sleep. Music helps during his waking hours. A Mozart CD called *Morning Meditation* is a favorite. He grunts a lot. Everything is an effort including walking, standing up, and sitting down.

2/25: 5:15 pm. "Who is going to win the race?" Edward asks.

"What race?" I ask.

"Aren't we waiting to hear about the race?" he says.

"There isn't any race," I say.

"Then what are we waiting for?"

"We're waiting for you to poop!" I say, injecting a bit of humor. "It's been three days."

As he gets into bed Edward says, "how long will I live? I want to go home."

"We are home," I say. "Where is home for you?"

"New York City," he says.

"That was forty years ago," I say.

"Tell them I need another blanket," he says.

Maybe he thinks this is a motel? I get another blanket and cover him. We have a ritual now at bedtime. We say the Lord's Prayer. Then I recite some Sanskrit prayers, do some reiki on his body.

When I kiss him goodnight, I say "I love you."

We look at each other as he says, "I love you too."

Each night of this ritual I wonder if this is our last kiss. How close to death is he? In my mind I feel 'the shadow of death' linger as I leave the room.

2/25: Before bed I ask, "Did you pee?"

"I already did!" he says, agitated. But I know he didn't. I say nothing. He goes into the bathroom, brushes his teeth and pees.

"You shouted at me that you had peed," I say, "that's not right."

"I'm sorry," he says, "but sometimes I can't control myself." This remark shows awareness of his illness and an admission that he hurt my feelings. It makes me feel recognized and valued. Apologies are unusual for Edward. He usually gets defensive.

3/5: This morning, around 8:00, I am in the kitchen when I hear a loud noise. Edward is on his knees in the bathroom, grasping the wicker bench with one hand and the toilet seat with the other. He says he got twisted around in his pants when he got up from the toilet and fell. He didn't hurt himself, but it scared us both. I now try to anticipate when he is in the bathroom so I can help him. His skin itches a lot, so I lather it with castor oil.

3/7: Edward weighs 134.8 lbs. naked and 140 with his clothes on after eating. He used to weigh 170 lbs. He has lost 10 lbs since seeing Dr. Friedman. I call her to report on his weight. I tell her that an echocardiogram would just increase Edward's anxiety. She says she will cancel the procedure and call Hospice of Hudson Valley to have

Edward evaluated. I feel like it's Christmas and I just received the greatest gift. Yes, I am sad because calling in Hospice is the prelude to the end of Edward's life, but he is suffering, and I need help. Now, that help is coming.

3/8: A Hospice nurse comes to examine Edward. Usually, if the patient qualifies for Hospice care, it indicates that he or she has six months to live. A patient can withdraw from Hospice and resume care depending on the course of the illness. Dementia is a common reason for admission to the multiple services that Hospice offers through Medicare. Edward qualifies. Dr. Friedman advises the Hospice nurse of his deteriorating symptoms, especially the weight loss. I am grateful for her input. After the nurse leaves, Edward is disoriented and nasty.

"You are f*cking things up," he says. "I want to sleep."

I turn on the TV to distract him. It's 5:00 pm. Maybe it's the sundown syndrome, but I think it is more than that.

"Something is wrong in this house!" he says, his agitation rising. Though Edward may not have known why the nurse was here – he dozed off most of the time – he is sensitive to what is happening around him. He may have picked up the vibrations associated with enrollment in Hospice care and what that means.

At supper, he imagines he has already eaten. "It's right over there, in a bag," he says, pointing to the fireplace. He's angry. He mistakes the floor for water and is hesitant to walk on it.

At night, he talks a lot in his sleep.

3/12: Around 9:00 am I go to the bathroom and see

feces on the braided rug, the floor, everywhere, as he sits on the toilet. He seems oblivious to the mess.

"This is it," I say angrily. "It's Depends, 24/7."

He says nothing. His eyes are vacant. I feel bad that I was angry.

"I'm sorry," I say. "Let me clean this first, then we will clean you."

He is pensive at supper. He complains of a stomachache. I wonder if there is a tumor.

"You have to help me. I'm worried about my life. I'm scared," he says.

"Of what?" I ask.

"Of no future, no meaning," he says.

3/13: Edward thinks we are on a trip. It is afternoon and he is sitting on the wing-back chair. He is very groggy. "I don't feel right," he says.

"Physically? Mentally? Emotionally?" I ask.

"Everything," he says. "All I know is I want to sleep. I'm cold."

I cover his legs with a throw.

3/14: During the night, Edward pees in his Depends. At breakfast, he can't distinguish between oatmeal, bread, and tea. I lead him to the living room where he meditates. I have a fire going. It snowed six inches last night.

Later, in the bathroom, he asks, "what am I doing now?"

"You're pulling up your pants," I say.

A Hospice volunteer has come twice this week so that I can go out shopping, knowing that Edward is in safe hands. Today it is a kindly older gentleman.

**

Last Days

In Plato's *Phaedo,* a dialogue takes place between Socrates and several of his friends, including Crito and Phaedo. It is the last day of Socrates' life. He is in prison, awaiting his death, after being convicted at trial of corrupting the Athenian youth with impious ideas. Socrates is amused by his friends' arguments that the law unjustly convicted him and that they will help him escape from prison. He argues that the true philosopher is in love with death of the body because it will facilitate the soul's release. For the soul to acquire pure knowledge and journey into immortality, says Socrates, it must not be disturbed by the body and bodily desires. The mind, which is the guide into the afterlife, needs to be clear, possessed of reason. When its light is veiled by the presence of the body, the flight of the soul into the light of truth is hampered. So, says Socrates, I welcome death. As he drinks the vial of poison, served to him reluctantly by the prison attendant, his last words to his friends are a request that they pay off a debt he owes someone. Socrates' detachment from the death of his body is exquisitely shown in this remark.

What happens to awareness at death? In Hindu Vedanta it is believed that the individual soul or *jiva,* as embodied Spirit or embodied Awareness, departs at the death of the body through the crown chakra at the top of the skull.

Chakras are subtle wheels of light energy located at seven principal sites in the physical body. The seventh chakra, or crown chakra, is the site of divine light and wisdom. At death, it is considered beneficial for someone to sit with the body and assist the soul in its departure by prayer and meditation. Tibetan Buddhists call the interim state of the soul as it leaves this world *bardo*. In the *Bhagavad Gita*, Krishna tells Arjuna: "The Spirit, which pervades all that we see, is imperishable. Nothing can destroy the Spirit.... As a man discards his threadbare robes and puts on new, so the Spirit throws off Its worn-out bodies and takes fresh ones." [95]

According to the doctrine of reincarnation – which Hinduism and Buddhism embrace – the soul continues its spiritual evolution in the next embodiment. Spiritual teachings on reincarnation tell us that we have died many times but the memory of living and dying in other bodies is not accessible to us. Greek mythology speaks of the river Lethe, one of the rivers in the underworld of Hades. Once crossed at death, the soul forgets its previous life. Judaism posits a belief in the soul, but the definition of an afterlife remains mysterious. After the burial of the body, family and friends gather to sit for seven days to mourn the deceased and contemplate God's presence in prayer. When asked in an interview whether he believed in an afterlife, Rabbi Abraham Joshua Heschel said: "Yes, we believe in an afterlife, but we have no information about it.... I think it's God's business what to do with me after life. Here, it's my business what to do with my life. So I leave it to Him." [96]

For Christians, the soul is sullied by sin and must undergo purification by faith and good works. The righteous soul journeys towards Christ consciousness in this world and the next. Dante portrays this journey as an ascent from purgatory to beatification in heaven. Reincarnation was a vital part of Christian doctrine until it was removed in 543 AD by Roman Emperor Justinian I. It was rejected again at the Second Council of Constantinople in 553 AD. In his book *Fear and Trembling*, philosopher Soren Kierkegaard describes the last breath of the faithful believer in Christ. The soul of this "knight of faith" has placed the love of God above any worldly happiness.[97] Therefore, says Kierkegaard,

A man can, in that last moment, concentrate his whole soul in a single glance towards the heaven from which all good gifts come and this glance is something that both he and the one he seeks understand; it means he has nevertheless remained true to his love.[98]

Edward's great love was his desire for Self-realization. He understood that spiritual evolution is the ultimate function of being born in human form. The attainment of a transcendent state of consciousness merges the soul into the force field of the Absolute or God. This process has many names in religious teachings, including self-realization, divine union, and enlightenment.

Edward liked to tell a story from the Hindu tradition which describes a devotee who prayed constantly for self-realization. He wanted to know how long it would take. One day, he received a visit from an angel of God. The angel pointed to a large tamarind tree. He said to the devotee, "Do you see the thousands of leaves on this tamarind tree? That is how many lifetimes it will take for you to achieve self-realization."

The angel expected the man to be downcast at this news. Instead, the devotee began to dance for joy.

"Are you not disappointed?" asked the angel.

"Oh, no," said the devotee. "I know now that I will be realized, however long it takes!"

At that voicing of the man's faith, God descended from heaven and entered the devotee as his own realized self.

According to Kübler-Ross, the last stage of the dying process is acceptance. People arrive at this stage in different ways. If a person has been allowed to express anger, cry in preparatory grief, and be in a supportive environment that helps him or her die with dignity, then the transition of separating from the body is made easier. It is natural in this last stage for the dying person to withdraw mentally and emotionally from the world. He or she loses interest in worldly activities, even ordinary acts like eating. The person prefers silence and does not readily engage in conversation. A certain passivity infuses and surrounds the person. There is often an absence of fear or despair. Kübler-Ross suggests that if the person can be brought to see, at the end of this life, that he or she has done his or her best to live a good life, then the circle of life can close in peace in the final moments.

One of the terminally ill patients in Kübler-Ross's care, a Mrs. W., was prepared to die. She was waiting for her husband to accept the fact of her imminent death. Mrs. W. was grateful for their marriage and their good life together, but it was time for her to leave him. Her husband refused to face this fact and insisted that she have an operation that might prolong her life. The operation was scheduled. As she was wheeled into the operating room, in great pain, she became wildly delusional, hallucinatory, and paranoid. The operation was canceled. She was wheeled back to her room where the delusions gradually ceased. Kübler-Ross discerned that there was in Mrs. W's psychotic episode an underlying awareness. Mrs. W. chose a logical strategy that enabled her to avoid the operation. After Kübler-Ross relayed to Mr. W. his wife's wish to die in peace and dignity, he finally accepted her impending death.

Before the age of hospitals, and the impersonal environment they embody, people died at home. The terminally ill were in a familiar environment where they felt safe, respected, and loved. Surrounded at their bedside by family and friends, they were cushioned from the fear and loneliness that can accompany the dying process. The Hospice movement arose as an effort to revive this traditional approach to death. Hospice was founded shortly after World War II when it was realized that giving attention to the care of the dying was an important, but missing, part of the medical profession. That care needed to include spiritual care. The work of Kübler-Ross was instrumental in the establishment of the Hospice movement which is now a global phenomenon.

The mission of Hospice's palliative care program is to help a person die at home with dignity and comfort, in the company of loving family members and friends. All life forms need love. Plants need love. Animals need love. People need love, even if – and especially if – they are sick. The human form, in its frailty, its mortality, asks for love to sustain its body in life and be present at the body's departure. The traditional format of Hospice care is augmented by accessibility to the new technologies and medicines that may help to make the transition at death less stressful. One of my good friends, who did not have Alzheimer's disease, but did have a terminal illness at age eighty-eight, received Hospice care when he returned home from his last trip to the hospital. When he was brought into his bedroom and placed in a hospital bed, he looked up at the ceiling. It was an A-framed ceiling with big cedar beams holding the structure in place. He grinned, and his face lit up in retelling the event. He said to me, "I looked up and I said out loud, 'this is my ceiling! I'm home!'" He died in his sleep a few days later.

Hospice provides numerous services: nursing care 24/7; equipment like walkers, shower chairs, and oxygen tanks, brought to one's home as needed; a box of medications that may be needed, with instructions; volunteers who enable the caregiver to leave the house for a few hours; social workers and chaplain care. Hospice even offers retreat facilities for caregivers so that they can have some respite from the constant care they have chosen to provide to their loved ones. Hospice serves the caregiver as well as the person who has a terminal illness. Hospice stays with patient and caregiver for the entire journey, as well as beyond through letters of consolation and bereavement services. The combination of empathy and efficiency was notable in all the Hospice personnel I met.

<u>Journal entries</u>

The following journal entries cover the last two weeks of Edward's life. A rapid decline is displayed, exacerbated by several falls.

3/17/2023: I must repeat everything as Edward either doesn't hear or doesn't comprehend the words. He sits on the sofa, with a fire blazing in the wood stove, and hallucinates.

"Where are those fires I put along the hallway?" he asks.

He thinks the living room is a bedroom. He says we need beds for all the people living here. I show him our bedroom.

"It's just us here," I say.

3/19: Getting up from the sofa, Edward falls on the rug; no injury. He weighs 131.8 lbs. in underwear. I feel that we are getting close to the end. I don't want him to suffer.

3/20: Edward sleeps until 1:00 pm. It's harder for him to walk. He only eats half of his cereal. At supper he says, "I don't feel right." Edward goes to bed early, 6:45. He uses his walker, especially at night. If he gets up to pee, I have to help him. We need to ask Hospice for a commode by the bed.

3/21: Edward is confused tonight at supper; he thinks the salad is cake. "I feel like my world is falling apart," he says. Is this a premonition of death? Undressing for bed, he can't tell the difference between trousers and socks. There's a lot of talking in his sleep, quasi dream-state, hallucinating, calling out. I put my hands on his shoulders to calm him. I try to remain a rock for him, though inside I feel like Jello.

3/25: At lunch he says, "I've lost my appetite. I feel strange, useless." I explain that he has family who care about him. He has no joy in eating.

3/26: "I'm tired of life," Edward says. He is very weak today; we hardly walk to the corner and back. It is warm for March. It is a treat sitting on the patio with him in the sun and meditating together.

3/27: Edward sleeps all day. I can't rouse him. He gets nasty when I try. I call his nurse Tim who suggests Haldol.

"Don't touch me," he says. "I want to rest, nothing to get up for."

Tim comes over and gets him to take Haldol with orange juice and water. He may be dehydrated.

At 5:00 pm I get him up for supper. "I don't feel right," he says. "Something is wrong with me."

"Where?" I ask.

"The middle," he says, pointing to his chest. He eats a little and then gets back in bed. We pray.

He says, before falling off to sleep, "I see a long line of cars." I immediately think of a funeral procession. I don't know how or when it will end but I feel heavy, weighed down with the knowledge that we are in the last days of Edward's life.

3/29: This is the second time Edward sleeps all day. James' wife Ronnie comes over. She brings a six-pack of Ensure and makes a milkshake in the blender, adding ice cream. She takes it to Edward. He is in bed, his head propped up with pillows. Later, I bring a tray to Edward: half a sandwich, orange slices and tea. He eats the meal. Afterwards, he gets up to pee, then goes back to bed. At 6:45 pm, he says he is thirsty. I give him orange juice. "The longer I live the more screwed up I feel," he says. "Can you help me?" I am touched by this request. I feel close to tears. I talk to him about what is most important to remember, that we are not the body, mind, or ego. We are God in embodied form. "We are really God," he says. I tell him I am going to fix his favorite dish, spaghetti, for supper. He eats at the table in his robe. At 8:00, he is back in bed. He says he is very cold. I cover him with an extra heavy wool blanket. He is hallucinating about 'going home.'

"We are home," I say. "This is your bed."

"Can I sleep here every night?" he asks.

"Yes," I say.

"Then I am satisfied," he says, managing a little smile. I well up.

He says his head feels hard. He wants me to massage it, which I do. He thinks it's George Washington's birthday. He's not hearing or comprehending well. He is in and out of reality.

"Do you know where your keys are?" he asks.

He's thirsty. I give him water. James comes over to read to his dad from a biography of Ramakrishna. He sits on the side of the bed and reads slowly. James and his family are leaving for Belize in a few days. It's spring break for his two sons. The timing is unfortunate, but I don't want to tell James to cancel his vacation. His dad could last several weeks. They will be back in twelve days. When I bend over to kiss Edward goodnight, I see a sunken, sallow face. The image of his young, handsome face rises in my mind – the disarming smile, the alluring hazel eyes. The two images clash.

Edward is delirious at night and very thirsty. He gets up to pee three times; I help him. He is very weak in the legs.

"I've been eating apples for three weeks," he says. "Where is that pitcher of coffee?" A shift has taken place. Maybe it's permanent. I can't sleep. I sit in the chair near the bed and meditate, for both of us. Acceptance of what is happening to Edward is not only his task; it is mine too. To offer no resistance, to remember the soul continues to live as the body dies. As the Bible says: "For everything there is a season, and a time to every purpose under the heaven: a time to be born, and a time to die...." [99] Remembering this verse and the simplicity of the meditation practice calms me. I get back into bed and fall asleep.

3/30: 5:00 pm Edward is very cold. He lies down on the bed. He says his stomach hurts. I put a heating pad on his stomach. I may give him a sedative later; it's in a box that Hospice gave me along with other medications. There is explosive diarrhea all over the bathroom floor and in his Depends.

3/30: Edward is having difficulty speaking. He can't formulate nor comprehend words. His words are jumbled. I think this condition, aphasia, signals more atrophy of the temporal and frontal regions, particularly Wernicke and Broca areas. Edward can't distinguish foods or feed himself. I am feeding him. He is using a walker now because his leg muscles are weak. The decline seems rapid. When we call his sister Dolores, I hear him trying to make a coherent sentence. He is slurring words. It's heartbreaking to see the man I love wither like autumn leaves. I try to see that it isn't the man that withers, it is his body.

3/31: Friday morning, downhill. He falls twice. The second time, while I am in the kitchen, I hear a loud crash. I run to the bedroom and see that, in getting out of bed, he fell on the wood floor and hit his head against the metal baseboard. He is frantic as we try unsuccessfully to get him to a standing position. His body is too heavy. I call Tim. He comes right over, lifts him up and puts him in bed. Edward is now bedridden. He may have hurt his leg or hip; we are not sure.

Pee goes into the Depends and out on the sheet. I help Tim lift Edward onto his side to clean him. Moving him appears to cause pain. Tim says he will order a hospital bed and commode. As Tim leaves, he suggests giving Edward a sedative later. I try to give him the sedative, but I can't lift his head and he doesn't have the strength to lift it himself. I start to panic. I call James and he reminds me to use more pillows behind Edward's head. I do that and then I can give him the sedative.

I am exhausted and constipated from stress. Lord help me. I am sorry I lost it. I apologize to Edward for panicking. I take his hand in mine. I lend the strength of my hand to his limp hand. Another Hospice nurse comes to evaluate his bodily injuries. She says he may have had a stroke. He is mumbling and hallucinating. I'm afraid the second fall has changed things for the worse.

4/2: It is Palm Sunday. John, his wife and two sons drive up to be with me. I call Hospice since Edward seems to be in pain. He is in bed, his eyes closed. Nurse Kate and an assistant arrive in the early afternoon. Kate is delightful: kind, calm, and competent. She introduces herself to Edward, then gives him a sedative to relax him (Lorazepam). Kate assesses his vital signs, then wipes his body with clean cloths and changes him into a new Depends.

"Does Edward have a favorite T-shirt?" she asks. I give

her a T-shirt which she cuts down the front. She puts it on him like a hospital gown. "We want to make him comfortable," she says, as she smooths the blankets around Edward's supine body.

Kate gives him a low dose of morphine for pain and shows me how to administer the dosage. Edward seems relaxed now. We all leave the room and go to the dining room where we sit down around the table. Kate explains that Edward is "actively dying."

"Dying is hard work," she says, "because the body resists and doesn't want to die." [100] This sounds like the instinct of self-preservation. Words from the *Bhagavad Gita* come to mind where Krishna explains to Arjuna that in this material world there is a "persistent clinging to life." [101]

"At most, he has a week," Kate says. I hope he passes sooner. I think this is what Edward wants, what he has been saying all along. Yet hearing this thought in my mind feels disobedient to God's will. I need to submit to the flow of events, whatever they are. I need to trust that Edward's soul will be guided out of the body at exactly the right time.

Kate says not to feed Edward or give him water. I am to use the sponge-like Q-tips Hospice provides to swab the inside of his mouth and keep it moist. After Kate and her assistant leave, John's wife Magda and I alternate sitting with Edward most of the day. John and his two sons are doing some outside work. I cook Indian food. We eat an early dinner together, but the sadness underneath is palpable. I am giving Edward meds at regular hours: a sedative and a low dose of morphine. I find our SONY tape recorder and alternate the playing of the Christian vespers service of Evensong and the Gayatri mantra to provide a continuum of serene background music.

Magda and I take turns holding Edward's hand. His breathing becomes noisy, rasping. Magda records a video of him on her phone. At one point, when I come into the bedroom, she is holding both his hands. His arms flail involuntarily. When I say, "I will sit with him now," there is an urgency to his flailing arms. He tries to raise his head and speak but he can't.

"He knows your voice," Magda says. As I sit on the bed and hold his hands, his arms moving, I sing the Gayatri in time with the tape recording. We are in silent communication through the music and the movement of our hands.

John and family leave for home around 8:00 pm. I take a shower around 10:00 and get in bed next to Edward. I hold his left hand. It is warm. He is breathing heavily; the sound is loud and raspy. I can't sleep. His hand is getting cool. I pull the blanket over his hands. It must be close to midnight when I drift off to sleep.

I don't know how long I sleep but I awaken with a start, look over, and see that he is not breathing. His mouth is open, his eyes closed, as they have been. I touch near his mouth and put my ear there. No breath. He is gone. I stay by the body and speak to him and pray over him until a Hospice nurse comes to pronounce the death of his body. It is 2:00 am. I call John and he says he is driving up. About an hour later, the funeral director and an assistant arrive. John arrives a few minutes later. He helps the funeral director and assistant roll the body into a bag. Edward's lifeless body rolls over stiff as a board. The soul no longer enlivens it. His soul left while I slept.

It is April 3rd, Monday morning, shortly after 3:00 am. As they take the body out the front door, I realize that I didn't hear the grandfather clock toll the hour with its pronounced gong. I go into the living room and see that the pendulum is still. The clock which Edward bought at an auction in New York City fifty years ago had stopped its faithful recording of time.

John stays over and spends the next day with me. We have trouble reaching James who is in Belize. When we finally get a phone connection, I tell him that his dad passed in the night. James is distraught because he wasn't present for his dad's death. I tell James not to feel guilty that he is not here because he has always been faithful to his dad. He met his dad's every need during his sickness.

"It is John's turn to be present at the last," I say.

To both sons I say, "Your dad lost interest in life. He couldn't connect to life anymore. He wanted to die and maybe through the serious fall it became possible." I told them that Edward's soul was ready to leave, but his body tried to hang on by labored breathing – a common sign that the end is near. Their dad's presence in this world was ending. His soul was now at rest in that space of mystery where our souls go to continue their journey.

***

Epilogue: **Gifts of Adversity**

<u>Journal entry</u>

It is Earth Day, April 22nd, 2023. We gather as a family to spread Edward's ashes around two young peach trees in the backyard. Our party includes James and his wife Ronnie, John and his wife Magda, and the four teenage grandsons – Mark, Adam, Jonah, and Eli. I read from the *Bhagavad Gita* as we take turns sprinkling the ashes. It feels surreal, standing there in a circle honoring Jadick (*grandfather* in Polish) with a box of gray ashes. This is all that is left of his body. We sing *Amazing Grace*. I invite everyone to say a few words to commemorate Edward's life. The teenagers are shy, but they murmur a loving goodbye to their grandfather.

After the ceremony we sit around the wicker table on the patio, recalling memories. James remembers how his dad, bare-chested in 88-degree weather, installed the radiant heat floor in James' new straw-bale house, fifteen years ago. John recalls how Edward changed the trajectory of his life during a difficult period in high school. He calls his dad "my savior". We remember with fondness Edward's quirky mannerisms. John and James do imitations; we all laugh. We remember Edward's amazing ability to recite passages from Shakespeare and Keats. I talk about qualities in Edward that I admire: his steadfast devotion to the truth, his mix of playfulness and seriousness, his love for me and his family, and his loyalty to The School – the place where we both grew as spiritual seekers. Our gathering gives some closure. It resuscitates the family unit, even as that unit is minus one important member.

***

With a terminal illness like Alzheimer's disease, the grief that accompanies the loss of a loved one starts a long time before the death of the body. A caregiver experiences it every day in some form. I experienced it for six years. When Edward died, I felt empty inside but empty also of tears. I didn't cry until several months passed. A conversation with my older son John triggered that searing moment. For three days I couldn't stop crying. I wrote a poem during that time. It seemed important to put on paper what I was experiencing, now that I lived alone.

LOSING A SPOUSE

It's in the small things

that you first feel the shrinkage.

Catching yourself saying *we*

instead of *I*,

setting the table for one,

buying too many groceries.

Your hand slides across the sheet

smooth and cool,

and empty.

But most of all

having to listen

to the blaring horns of silence

that echo in every room.

John and James said that when the feeling of loss was still raw, they would often find themselves tearing up. When we gathered at Thanksgiving, seven months after Edward's death, James was offering a prayer at the table when he suddenly broke down. It was the first holiday in which Edward was not present. Since that time, both sons have supported me with calls and invitations to supper. Holidays can be particularly painful because of the memories attached to them. The experience of loss lingers. It must be given its time.

The pain of trauma and of loss is balanced to some extent by the gifts that adversity bestows. One such gift is the strengthening of family ties around the core of loss. Death is a rite of passage, a transition from one state to another. It signals a sudden stop in the business of ordinary life. We, as a family and community, stop to commemorate someone special, in an atmosphere outside linear time. The time of mourning the loss of a loved one is what anthropologist Victor Turner calls a *liminal phase*. The word *liminal* is from the Latin *"limen"* which means *threshold*. It is an uncertain time of transition between the leaving of what is familiar and the beginning of a new phase of life. There is no time limit on how long this experience of liminality lasts. It is a time of waiting, not knowing what you are waiting for, except that you need relief from the feeling of being displaced. Relationships within the family and close friends are intensified to counteract this feeling. The frequent disorientation that Edward felt as an effect of Alzheimer's disease is not unlike the feeling I experienced when he died: feeling that I had lost contact with the ground beneath my feet, feeling lost in my own home. For many native peoples, the person who dies is still part of a greater whole – the tribe. The elders of the community are especially valued for their wisdom, hewn from experience. When they die, their lives are celebrated. They become revered ancestors and are still considered members of the tribe. I want to think of Edward in this way, still part of our tribe of family and close friends.

Those left behind by the death of a loved one seek spiritual comfort. For me, meditation and prayer were essential modes of healing. The experience of feeling my way towards emotional adjustment to the loss of my husband continues. As time passes, time also gradually covers the wound. I think of the Boswellia tree, which grows in the dry regions of Africa, India, and the Middle East. It secretes a type of resin when it is injured. The oil of that resin is frankincense. The tree uses resin to cover the wound so that, as healing takes place from within, the wounded area is protected from exterior forces. In the same way, when a loved one is ill and dies, the heart is wounded. It needs to heal. Emotions are raw and tender. Family and friends cover the wounded heart with love. That love and spiritual practice become the frankincense of healing.

The lessons which terminal illness provides are also a gift. In Alzheimer's disease, the deterioration of the brain is a slow but chronic phenomenon that can last up to twenty years. There is plenty of time for the person undergoing the illness and the caregiver to taste its bitter fruit but also to listen to the silent teaching that the breakdown of the body is imparting. Illness is a teacher. Illness is the flip side of health, with an equal role to play in one's life. It is not an aberration. By its means we find out about the whole of ourselves. The suffering body holds both our personal history and our collective history as human beings. By acceptance of illness, even terminal illness, we open ourselves to understanding that history. We open ourselves to the healing energy of the universe.

Because one of the first signs of Alzheimer's disease is the atrophying of the temporal lobes – particularly the hippocampus where present meets past in memories – the practice of mindfulness, of presence, is the foremost vehicle of communion, as well as the premier exercise for the decaying brain. The caregiver practices mindfulness and encourages the loved one to practice it too. This practice is a gift. When Edward lost his short-term memory, communication was confined to the moment. Every moment that we remembered to be present to each other in love was precious.

As the disease advanced, we were continually asked to assent to whatever presented itself. When we were able to accept the daily drama of living with Alzheimer's disease, I believe our souls were strengthened in compassion and courage. Perhaps illness of the body is the effort by the soul to instruct us about who we are and who we are not. By breaking down barriers in the subconscious and dredging up old ideas and beliefs about ourselves and each other, Alzheimer's disease dared Edward and me to self-examine and, also, to reimagine our relationship. We needed to keep it from deteriorating under stress. Illness was laying upon both of us burdens which we needed to transmute into gifts. I needed to learn the virtues of patience and selflessness in service to Edward. These were heavy gifts to unwrap, but sometimes they broke through the crust of self-concern and the weight of responsibility. I can't say for sure what Edward was learning but it may be the virtue of surrender. Compliance with what is may be the hardest human task, and the most courageous one.

During those six years of caring for Edward, I had to remember that even though Edward's brain was fragmenting into pieces of itself, he was still aware. He was still experiencing the dying process. The knowledge that awareness is not limited to the brain but suffuses the whole mind-body, that awareness is a constant, not a variable, is another gift. As Edward's illness progressed, the conviction that his soul, alive in awareness, would not be contaminated by the physical assault on his brain grew ever stronger. It emerged like sunlight from the clouds to remind me of its authority. It appeared at odd times, as evidenced in the philosophy class Edward conducted four months before he died. Awareness is the quality of the present moment. Our minds may leave the awareness of awareness, through distraction, but we can always return to it through reawakening into the present moment.

As a caregiver, I came to understand that for the person facing a terminal illness, life's meaning is whittled down to what has been most important. Discover that and the person comes alive, for what is precious is remembered the longest. The veil of forgetting is just a veil. There is great wealth behind the veil. The caregiver does her or his best to discover and present to the loved one this wealth. For Edward it was meditation and family. And, for all of us, it is the treasured memory of those family members and friends whose hearts are bound to ours in love. Love is the constant that preserves the humanity of both the person living with Alzheimer's disease and the caregiver. Love connects the two souls. Love flows like a river if we swim in it.

As I now approach the second anniversary of Edward's passing, I am buoyed by the belief that each of us is here on earth to express the Eternal Spirit in embodied form. We are here to live and model the virtues of Spirit and help others to do the same. This is our filial duty, our main function as *homo sapiens*, 'that being that knows' – how to live. There are those, including myself, who believe that at death the soul retires for a time to another plane or dimension of reality. It then returns to earth to continue its evolution towards divine union or Self-realization. This was Edward's aim in life – to strive for Self-realization. But even if this presumption of reincarnation isn't true, our lives can still have meaning. To strive for perfection is no small thing. It is the work of the saints. If one strives to attain all the virtues, especially love for God and neighbor, then, says St. Teresa of Avila, "even if the whole world deafen you with its cries, what matter, so long as you are in the arms of God?"[102]

Appendix I: Loving Kindness Meditation [103]

1. Find a quiet place to sit and connect your heart to basic goodness and love....

2. Bring to mind a time when you were happy. Recall the place and the people around you. Let the happiness that you felt then be renewed in your heart. Let it fill you completely. Now speak or repeat in mind: "May I be happy, may I be healthy, may I live in peace." Rest within this serene, unburdened feeling for a few moments.

3. Bring to mind someone who is dear to you. Visualize his or her face. Recall a time when you were happy together. Let loving kindness fill your heart and be extended to this person. Now speak or repeat in mind: "May you be happy, may you be healthy, may you live in peace." Rest within this feeling for a few moments.

4. Bring to mind a person (it may be the same person visualized in #3) with whom you experienced a difficult situation that momentarily disrupted the relationship between you and this person. Recognize the humanity and the spiritual essence of this person. Let loving kindness fill your heart. Speak or repeat in mind: "May you be happy, may you be healthy, may you live in peace." Rest within this feeling for a few moments.

5. Radiate loving kindness to all beings, especially those who are suffering from mental or physical illness. Speak or repeat in mind: "May everyone, everywhere, be happy, healthy, and may they live in peace." Rest in silence for a few moments.

Appendix II: Two Poems

The 'A' Word

Uncensored tongue

spews words unkind;

don't react, she thinks,

let them pass through you.

She learns to be quiet

and, most times,

receives in silence

the infrequent blow.

He doesn't remember their dialogue

of two minutes ago.

"How old am I?" he asks.

"88," she says.

"When do we go home?" he asks.

"We are home," she says.

"What should I wear?" – and then

"No, don't tell me what to do!"

She backs off.

Routines get mixed up in his mind;

she helps him sort things out,

tries not to be 'the teacher.'

"Do I shower now, or eat?"

"How old am I anyhow?"

"88," she says.

She knows he is not the cellular rot in his brain;

she needs to remember how they were before.

"Where do I sleep tonight?" he asks.

"Here, with me," she says,

turning down the covers.

"Are we married?" he asks.

She looks up, startled,

then smiles.

"54 years," she says. They both laugh.

She turns out the light.

"I love you," he says,

pressing his hand on hers.

"I love you too," she says,

as the tears come.

First Aid

The robin takes her evening bath

in the little pond,

fluttering her feathers

amidst water hyacinths

and fallen dogwood petals;

the image,

for the moment,

sutures the grief,

with a smile.[104]

About The Author

Lyla graduated Phi Beta Kappa from the University of North Carolina, Chapel Hill, with a BA in English and Drama. While engaged in an early career in the theatre she met Edward, a fellow actor. The two married and moved into a brownstone on Manhattan's west side. Edward turned to his carpentry skills to make a living while Lyla became the mother of two sons. They found a spiritual home at the School of Practical Philosophy in New York City where they studied and taught philosophy and meditation. It wasn't until their sons were grown and out on their own that Lyla revisited academia. She earned a Ph.D. in Anthropology at the State University of New York/Albany and taught courses in anthropology and religious studies for 18 years at the college level.

Since her retirement, Lyla has been presenting courses at lifelong learning centers at college campuses in the Hudson Valley. Lyla is a reiki master with training in shamanic healing. She received professional training in mindfulness-based stress-reduction (MBSR) from Jon Kabat-Zinn. Lyla has written two books. The first, *Pause Now: Handbook for a Spiritual Revolution* (2009), describes the spiritual practice of pausing – an exercise in sensory awareness. Lyla teaches that pausing helps us stay in the present moment where life is taking place. Only in the moment can we learn how to release our talents for the welfare of the community and the world. The second book, *Homesick: Finding Our Way Back to a Healthy Planet* (2018), explains the origins of global warming and offers solutions based in ecological sustainability. Lyla was inspired to write *Homesick* by the students in her ecological anthropology course. Lyla is also an accomplished poet. Her poetry has appeared in Chronogram magazine.

When Lyla's husband of 54 years of marriage died of Alzheimer's disease almost two years ago, she felt compelled to write a book that might be of help to fellow caregivers. Lyla was Edward's sole caregiver for six years. It was a difficult experience. But difficult experiences can yield important lessons.

Her new book, *My Years as an Alzheimer's Caregiver: Transcending Loss by Nurturing Spirit*, traces the journey she and her husband took through the labyrinth of Alzheimer's disease. The book's approach is unique. It weaves together three elements: first, a scientific description of the normal brain and how it becomes disfigured by the toxic proteins that define Alzheimer's disease; second, a spiritual teaching embodied in the mystical heart of religions that declares the soul to be untouched by the physical breakdown of the body; and third, an experiential component that brings to life through daily journal entries the progression of the disease and how the soul of the loved one can be nourished, even as the body fails.

To find out more about Lyla's work as an author and teacher visit **www.lylayastion.com**.

Notes

[1] The *Vedas* are the major Hindu scriptures. The Sanskrit root of the word *veda* is *veid* which is a verb meaning *to see*, or *to know*. One who knows the truth is a seer. *A-dvaita* means *not-two*. In Advaita Vedanta one seeks to know by direct experience the reality of Oneness.

[2] *King James Bible,* Luke 17:21

[3] *The Geeta*, trans. Shri Purohit Swami (London: Faber and Faber, 1965), p.60. The *Bhagavad Gita* is considered the jewel of the Hindu Upanishads. These scriptures were first heard as the revealed word *(shruti)* by seers of old who taught them orally before they were written down around 1500 BCE.

[4] In Hindu Vedanta the Self is interchangeably used with the words God and Spirit to denote divinity. The Sanskrit word *Brahman* translates as God. The individual soul, *Atman*, is equated in its realized state with Brahman.

[5] Rick Hanson, *Hardwiring Happiness*: *The New Brain Science of Contentment, Calm, and Confidence* (New York: Harmony Books, 2016), p.32.

[6] Elliott Ash et al., "Mindfulness reduces information avoidance", *Economic Letters*, March 2023, vol 224.
https://neurosciencenews.com/meditation-cognitive-bias-23372/

[7] In Chapter 2, mind will be defined as that which witnesses, guides, and imbues the brain with awareness and intelligence.

[8] Thich Nhat Hanh, *you are here, Discovering the Magic of the Present Moment* (Boulder, CO.: Shambhala, 2010), p.12.

[9] *King James Bible*, Matthew 18:20.

[10] Namenda is a receptor of glutamate, a neurotransmitter in the brain that facilitates synaptic functioning so that memories can be formed. Aricept is an acetylcholinesterase inhibitor. It prevents the breakdown of the neurotransmitter acetylcholine which assists communication between neurons and the muscles of the body so that motor coordination is efficient.

[11] See Shazia Vegar Siddiqui, Ushri Chatterjee, Devvarta Kumar, and Nishant Goval, "Neuropsychology of prefrontal cortex", *Indian Journal of Psychiatry*, 2008 Jul-Sep; 50(3), pp.202-208.
https://www.ncbi.nih.gov/pmc/articles/PMC2738354/?report

[12] See Ho Namkung, Sun-Hong Kim, and Akira Sawa, "The insula: an underestimated brain area in clinical neuroscience, psychiatry and

neurology", *Trends in Neuroscience* Apr 2017: 40(4), pp.200-207. https://pubmed.ncbi.nlm.nih.gov/28314446/

[13] From notes taken on 7/29/23 in conversation with Michael.

[14] See Oliver Sacks, *Awakenings* (New York: HarperPerennial, 1990), pp.60-61.

[15] See Marti Colom-Cadena, Caitlin Davis, Sonia Sirisi et al. "Synaptic oligomeric tau in Alzheimer's Disease – A potential culprit in the spread of tau pathology through the brain." *Neuron*, May 15, 2023, vol. 111 (13), pp.2170-2183. https://www.cell.com/neuron/fulltext/S0896-6273(23)

[16] **See** https://scitechdaily.com/stanford-reverses-cognitive-decline-in-alzheimers-with-brain-metabolism-drug/

[17] See Haoshen Shi, Yosef Koronyo, and Dieu-Trang Fuchs et al. "Retinal arterial Aβ40 deposition is linked with tight junction loss and cerebral amyloid angiopathy in MCI and AD patients." *Alzheimer's & Dementia*, 11 May 2023, vol 19 (11), pp.5185-5197. https://pubmed.ncbi.nlm.nih.gov/37166032

[18] See Aura Ferreiro, Joohee Choi, Jian Ryou et al. "Gut microbiome composition may be an indicator of preclinical Alzheimer's disease." *Science Translational Medicine*, 14 June 2023, vol. 15 (700). https://www.ncbi.nlm.nih.gov/pmc/articles/PMC1068

[19] *King James Bible*, Matthew 5:16.

[20] Neuroimmunology is a field of science which studies the interactions between two complex systems in the body: the nervous system and the immune system.

[21] Richard Geldard, *Anaxagoras and Universal Mind* (New York: Ralph Waldo Emerson Institute Books, 2007), p.24.

[22] *The Geeta*, trans. Shri Purohit Swami (London: Faber and Faber, 1965), p.60.

[23] Rabindranath Tagore, *Stray Birds* (New York: The Macmillan Company, 1916), p.4.

[24] *New International Version of the Bible* (NIV), 2 Corinthians 4:18.

[25] Rabindranath Tagore, *Stray Birds* (New York: The Macmillan Company, 1916), p.30.

[26] *The Ten Principal Upanishads*, trans. Shree Purohit Swami and W.B. Yeats (London: Faber and Faber, 1970), p.19.

[27] Rick Hanson, *Hardwiring Happiness: The New Brain Science of Contentment, Calm, and Confidence* (New York: Harmony Books, 2016), pp.41-44.

[28] Rick Hanson and Richard Mendius, *Buddha's Brain: the practical neuroscience of happiness, love and wisdom* (Los Angeles, New Harbinger Publications, 2009), p.7.

[29] Rick Hanson and Richard Mendius, *Buddha's Brain*, p.187.

[30] Daniel J. Siegel, *mind, a journey to the heart of being human* (New York: W.W. Norton & Company, 2017). Siegel's terms for mind and its extensions – *mindscape, mindsight*, and *mindsphere* – are described in this book.

[31] See Oliver Sacks, *The Man Who Mistook His Wife For A Hat* (New York: Vintage Books, 1985), p.234.

[32] *The Geeta*, trans. Shri Purohit Swami (London: Faber and Faber, 1965), p.60.

[33] *The Geeta*, trans. Shri Purohit Swami, p.59.

[34] *The Geeta,* trans. Shri Purohit Swami, p.59.

[35] *King James Bible*, Romans 8:22.

[36] Ralph Waldo Emerson, *Nature, Addresses and Lectures* in *Complete Works of Ralph Waldo Emerson* (Boston: Houghton-Mifflin, 1903), p.10.

[37] *The Geeta*, trans. Shri Purohit Swami (London: Faber and Faber, 1965), p.59.

[38] *Ten Principal Upanishads*, trans. Shree Purohit Swami and W.B. Yeats (London: Faber and Faber, 1970), p.38.

[39] *The Essential Rumi*, trans. Coleman Barks with John Moyne, A.J. Arberry, Reynold Nicholson (New York: Harper SanFrancisco, 1996), p.142. From the poem 'Childhood Friends.' © Coleman Barks. Used by permission of Coleman Barks.

[40] See Jacques Lusseyran, *And There Was Light* (Novato, CA: New World Library, 2014).

[41] *The Geeta*, trans. Shri Purohit Swami (London: Faber and Faber, 1965), p.59.

[42] *The Works of William Shakespeare* (Roslyn N.Y.: Walter J. Black, Inc., 1937), *Hamlet*, Act I, Scene 5, p.45.

[43] See Helane Wahbeh, Dean Radin, Cedric Cannard and Arnaud Delorme, "What if consciousness is not an emergent property of the brain? Observational and empirical challenges to materialistic models," *Frontiers in Psychology*, 02 September 2022. https://www.ncbi.nlm.nih.gov/pmc/articles/PMC9490

[44] See Helane Wahbeh et al. "What if consciousness is not an emergent property of the brain? Observational and empirical challenges to materialistic models."

[45] *The Geeta*, trans. Shri Purohit Swami (London, Faber and Faber, 1965), p.58.

[46] Dante, *The Divine Comedy 1: Hell*, trans. Dorothy L. Sayers (London: Penguin Books, 1949), p.85. Reproduced by permission of David Higham Associates.

[47] *The Geeta*, trans. Shri Purohit Swami (London: Faber and Faber, 1965), p.30.

[48] *The Geeta*, trans. Shri Purohit Swami (London: Faber and Faber, 1965), p.47.

[49] See Gretchen Reynolds, "Physical Activity and Aging Brains." *The New York Times*, 7 December 2021.

[50] Edward Bliss Reed, ed. *Shakespeare's Sonnets*. (New Haven: Yale University Press, 1923, 1961), p.73.

[51] This sequence of interrelated parts is called the hypothalamic-pituitary-adrenal axis (HPAA)

[52] *Rumi: In the Arms of the Beloved,* trans. Jonathan Star (New York: Jeremy P. Tarcher-Putnam, 2000), p.29. Copyright © 1997 by Jonathan Star. Used by permission of Jonathan Star and Tarcher, an imprint of Penguin Publishing Group, a division of Penguin Random House LLC. All rights reserved.

[53] See Zahinoor Ismail. Byron Creese, Dag Aarsland et al. (2022). "Psychosis in Alzheimer disease – mechanisms, genetics and therapeutic opportunities." *Nature Reviews Neurology* 18, pp.131-144. https://www.nature.com/articles/s41582-021-00597-3 . Another umbrella term for neuropsychiatric symptoms (NPS) is BPSD – behavioral and psychological symptoms of dementia.

[54] See L. Gurin. and S. Blum (2017). "Delusions and the Right Hemisphere: A Review of the Case for the Right Hemisphere as a Mediator of Reality-Based Belief." *The Journal of Neuropsychiatry*, 28 March 2017. Published online: https://dol.org/10.1176/appi.neruopsych.16060118

[55] William Shakespeare, *The Tragedy of Hamlet, Prince of Denmark*, Act 3, Scene 2 (New Haven: Yale University Press, 1947), pp.86-87.

[56] *The Geeta*, trans. Shri Purohit Swami (London: Faber and Faber, 1965), p.59.

[57] Joseph Campbell, *The Power of Myth* (New York: Anchor Books, 1991), p.146.

[58] Louis Untermeyer, ed. *The Book of Living Verse*. (New York: Harcourt, Brace and Company, 1945), p.300.

[59] See Mihaly Csikszentmihalyi, *Flow: The Psychology of Optimal Experience* (New York: HarperPerennial, 1990).

[60] *Writings from the Philokalia on Prayer of the Heart*, trans. E. Kadloubovsky & G.E.H. Palmer. (London: Faber and Faber,1975), p.250. Used with permission of Faber and Faber.

[61] See Oliver Sacks, *The Man Who Mistook His Wife for a Hat*. (New York: Vintage Books, 1985), p.269.

[62] From notes taken on 9/2/23 in conversation with Rev. Diane Epstein.

[63] From notes taken on 6/19/23 in conversation with David.

[64] William Shakespeare, *Merchant of Venice*, Act 5, Scene 1 (New Haven: Yale University Press, 1947), p.88.

[65] William Shakespeare, *Twelfth Night or What You Will*, Act 1, Scene 1 (New Haven: Yale University Press, 1947), p.1.

[66] In 2020, the most comprehensive study so far in assessing the value of music in treatment of dementia was conducted at the Betty Irene Moore School of Nursing at UC Davis. 4,107 residents in 265 nursing homes in CA. were given the personalized music playlists for listening on their iPods. The study revealed a decrease in the need for antipsychotic and anti-anxiety drugs, 13 per cent and 17 per cent respectively. Episodes of depression and aggression also decreased. Researchers concluded that the Music & Memory program awakened and nourished patients. It provides a gateway to transcend the sense of confinement, limitation, and loss imposed by Alzheimer's and other dementia diseases.

[67] See Katherine Carroll Britt, Jung Kwak, Gayle Acton, Kathy C. Richards, Jill Hamilton, & Kavita Radhakrishnan. 01 September 2022. "Measures of Religion and Spirituality in dementia: an integrative review." *Alzheimer's & Dementia: Translational Research & Clinical Interventions* /Volume 8, Issue 1. https://alzjournals.onlinelibrary.wiley.com

[68] Religious belief and practice are usually associated with traditional, formal religions – their scriptures, institutions, and rituals. Spirituality refers to a more expansive, individualized search for meaning that is found outside of religious institutions – in nature, for example, or in spiritual writings that elicit a feeling of the divine and the sacred.

[69] From notes taken on 9/2/23 in conversation with Rev. Diane Epstein.
[70] From notes taken on 9/2/23 in conversation with Rev. Diane Epstein.
[71] The Chinese religions of Confucianism and Taoism combine mind with heart. Confucius defined the individual person as *hsin* which means *mind-heart*. The self of the person (*hsin*) is a set of relationships (*li*); that is, the individual is seen as part of a continuum of relationships – family, community, nation, and all life. This integration of mind and heart fits the recent recognition in Western neuroscience of emotional intelligence as a valid type of intelligence – just different from the analytical, reasoning capacity traditionally associated with intelligence. Psychologist Robert Sternberg proposes a triarchic theory of intelligence. In his theory, intelligence has three aspects: analytical, creative, and practical (applying one's abilities to life situations).
[72] The School received a mantra meditation from the late Shantananda Saraswati, the Shankaracharya of the northern seat in India. The founder of the School of Practical Philosophy, Mr. Leon MacLaren, formed a relationship with the Shankaracharya who was considered a realized man. He passed on to Mr. MacLaren the teaching of Advaita Vedanta. Their conversations became the major material for classes at the School.
[73] Sanskrit is the language of Hindu Vedanta. The Sanskrit word for pure intellect is *buddhi*. The word for discursive mind (that which tends to get distracted by thoughts that take us away from the present moment) is *manas*.
[74] See Eileen Luders, Arthur W. Toga, Natasha Lapore, and Christian Gaser, "The underlying anatomical correlates of long-term meditation: Larger hippocampal and frontal volumes of gray matter," *NeuroImage*, 15 April 2009, vol 45 (3), pp.672-678.
https://www.ncbi.nlm.nih.gov/pmc/articles/PMC3184
[75] See Eileen Luders, Paul M. Thompson, Florian Kurth, et al., "Global and regional alterations of hippocampal anatomy in long-term meditation practitioners," *Human Brain Mapping*, December 2013, vol 34 (12), pp.3369-3375. https://pubmed.ncbi.nlm.nih.gov/22815233
[76] Jean Klein, *Living Truth*, ed. Emma Edwards (St. Peter Port, Guernsey, C. I.: Third Millennium Publications, 1995), p.96. Used by permission of Emma Edwards, president of the Jean Klein Foundation.
[77] See Adam Frank, "Scientists Found Ripples in Space and Time And You Have to Buy Groceries", *The Atlantic*, 29 July 2023.

[78] See Richard Gerber, M.D., *Vibrational Medicine* (Rochester, VT.: Bear & Company, 2001), pp.522-523.

[79] See Mitchell L. Gaynor, M.D., *The Healing Power of Sound: Recovery from Life-Threatening Illness Using Sound, Voice and Music* (Boston: Shambhala, 2002).

[80] See Benedict Carey, "Firing Up the Neural Symphony," *The New York Times*, 21 May 2019.

[81] See Pam Belluck, "Could Lights and Sounds Help People With Alzheimer's? They Worked in Mice", *The New York Times*, 15 March 2019, A18.

[82] From notes recorded at a seven-day Professional Training in Mindfulness-Based Stress Reduction,7-14 June, 2002, Omega Institute, Rhinebeck NY.

[83] See Appendix 1 for loving kindness meditation instructions.

[84] See Center for Mindfulness Studies, Toronto; American Mindfulness Research Association.

[85] Gamma waves induce connectivity between different regions of the brain leading to enhanced learning, memory, accurate information processing, and emotional balance. Gamma waves may have a positive effect in producing a cognitively coherent and unified perception of self and the world. Studies have linked abnormal gamma wave activity with neuroinflammation to pathological conditions of the central nervous system such as Alzheimer's disease, Parkinson's disease, and schizophrenia. There is evidence that gamma entrainment, using sensory stimulation, can protect neural networks. In experiments with mice who have AD, there is evidence that gamma entrainment improved cognitive and spatial memory. See Ao Guan, Shaoshuang Wang, Ailing Huang et al. "The role of gamma oscillations in central nervous system diseases: Mechanism and treatment." *Frontiers in Cellular Neuroscience*, 29 July 2022 vol 16. https://www.frontiersin.org/articleS/10.3389/fncel.2022.962957/full

[86] *King James Bible*, Matthew 18:21-35.

[87] William Shakespeare, *The Tragedy of Hamlet, Prince of Denmark*, Act 3, Scene 4. (New Haven: Yale University Press, 1947), p.115.

[88] Samuel H. Dresner, ed. *I Asked for Wonder: A Spiritual Anthology, Abraham Joshua Heschel* (New York: The Crossroad Publishing Company, 1999), p.22. Copyright © Abraham Joshua Heschel. Reprinted by arrangement with The Crossroad Publishing Company. https://www.crossroadpublishing.com

[89] *The Geeta*, trans. Shri Purohit Swami (London: Faber and Faber, 1965), P.44.

[90] From notes taken on 6/19/23 in conversation with David.

[91] From notes taken on 7/29/23 in conversation with Michael.

[92] From notes taken on 6/19/23 in conversation with David.

[93] From notes taken on 7/29/23 in conversation with Michael.

[94] From notes taken on 9/2/23 in conversation with Reverend Diane Epstein

[95] *The Geeta*, trans. Shri Purohit Swami (London: Faber and Faber, 1965), p.14.

[96] From "A conversation with Dr. Abraham Joshua Heschel", moderator NBC correspondent Carl Stern, Eternal Light program on NBC in association with The Jewish Theological Seminary, 1972.

[97] Soren Kierkegaard, *Fear and Trembling*, trans. Alastair Hannay (London: Penguin Books, 1985), p.68.

[98] Soren Kierkegaard, *Fear and Trembling*, p.78.

[99] *King James Bible*, Ecclesiastes 3:1-2.

[100] From notes taken on 4/2/23 of Nurse Kate's evaluation of Edward's condition.

[101] *The Geeta*, trans. Shri Purohit Swami (London: Faber and Faber, 1965), p.58.

[102] St. Teresa of Avila, *The Way of Perfection,* trans. E. Allison Peers (Mineola, NY: Dover Publications, Inc., 2012), p.121.

[103] This meditation is an adaptation of the loving kindness meditation described and taught by Buddhist teacher, Sharon Salzberg. Sources consulted were Sharon Salzberg's book, *Loving Kindness: The Revolutionary Art of Happiness* (Boulder: Shambhala, 2020) and the YouTube Tricycle 10-minute loving kindness meditation with Sharon Salzberg, https://www.youtube.com/watch?v=e-TeW9C10bc Retrieved 9/1/24, 7:45 PM.

[104] The two poems, *The 'A' Word* and *First Aid,* were written by Lyla Yastion. They appeared in Chronogram magazine in 2023.

Made in United States
North Haven, CT
11 July 2025

70534668R00173